Basic Guide to
Oral Health Education and Promotion

T0340686

BASIC GUIDE TO ORAL HEALTH EDUCATION AND PROMOTION

Third Edition

Alison Chapman

RDH, FAETC

Simon H. Felton

BSc (Hons)

WILEY Blackwell

Registered Offices
John Wiley & Sons, Inc., 111 River Street, Hoboken, NJ 07030, USA
John Wiley & Sons Ltd, The Atrium, Southern Gate, Chichester, West Sussex, PO19 8SQ, UK

Editorial Office
9600 Garsington Road, Oxford, OX4 2DQ, UK
For details of our global editorial offices, customer services, and more information about Wiley products visit us at www.wiley.com.

Wiley also publishes its books in a variety of electronic formats and by print-on-demand. Some content that appears in standard print versions of this book may not be available in other formats.

Library of Congress Cataloging-in-Publication Data

Names: Chapman, Alison, 1959- author. | Felton, Simon, 1970- author. | Preceded by (work): Felton, Ann. Basic guide to oral health education and promotion.
Title: Basic guide to oral health education and promotion / Alison Chapman, Simon H. Felton.
Other titles: Basic guide to dentistry series.
Description: Third edition. | Hoboken, NJ : Wiley-Blackwell, 2021. | Series: Basic guide dentistry series | Preceded by Basic guide to oral health education and promotion / Ann Felton, Alison Chapman, Simon Felton. Second edition. 2014. | Includes bibliographical references and index.
Identifiers: LCCN 2020026982 (print) | LCCN 2020026983 (ebook) | ISBN 9781119591627 (paperback) | ISBN 9781119591597 (adobe pdf) | ISBN 9781119591702 (epub)
Subjects: MESH: Health Education, Dental–methods | Health Promotion–methods | Oral Health–education | Dental Assistants
Classification: LCC RK60 (print) | LCC RK60 (ebook) | NLM WU 113 | DDC 617.6/0233–dc23
LC record available at https://lccn.loc.gov/2020026982
LC ebook record available at https://lccn.loc.gov/2020026983

Cover Design: Wiley
Cover Image: Paul Chapman

Set in 10/12.5pt Sabon by SPi Global, Pondicherry, India
Printed and bound by CPI Group (UK) Ltd, Croydon, CR0 4YY

C9781119591627_141023

Dedication

Love your patients and they will do anything that you ask.

Ann Felton (1942–2007)

Ann Felton made patients smile and their smiles brighter. Ann was a dental hygienist, tutor, mentor, and writer; a wife to David, and a mother to Sarah and Simon. She also ran her own oral health education course for dental nurses who she referred to as 'the darlings of dentistry'.

Ann wrote the first edition of this book in difficult circumstances, yet retained her love of the subject and her wonderful sense of humour throughout. This third edition is dedicated to Ann's life and work.

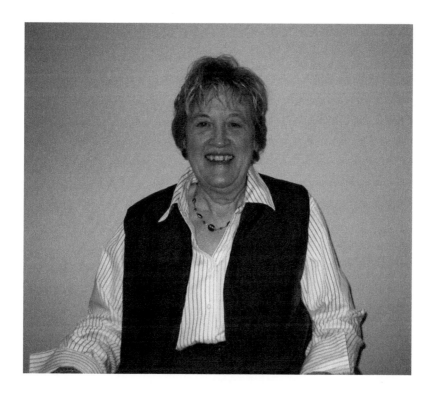

Contents

Foreword

This third edition of the *Basic Guide to Oral Health Education and Promotion* will be welcomed by dental care professionals (DCPs).

The first edition (2008) was a collaboration between two very experienced oral health educators and dental hygienists, Ann Felton and Alison Chapman, and editor Simon Felton who (together with practice manager Elizabeth Hill), ran a very successful oral health education course for over 10 years. A revised second edition was updated by Alison and Simon (both now e-learning course consultants), and published in 2014. It was dedicated to the life and work of Ann who sadly died in 2007 following a brave struggle with breast cancer.

There are very few books published in the UK that have been created by DCPs for DCPs, and this book is a perfect model, having been written with the experience and insight that comes from a lifetime of tutoring on the subject and working closely with other professionals and patients. This has given the authors a comprehensive understanding of the needs of students and practitioners in delivering oral health education and promotion.

Healthcare professionals have long been aware of the need to regularly update their knowledge and skills in this era of fundamental change and development. Accordingly, the authors have comprehensively reviewed and updated this edition, encompassing the many changes that have been brought about in dentistry, through advances in scientific research, technology, products, and policy.

The book takes the reader on a carefully thought-out journey, beginning with the underpinning knowledge that is vital to students and newcomers to oral health education, and is a welcome revision aid for all the dental team. Each chapter has been reviewed and updated. For example, Chapter 4 includes the BSP 2017 Classification of Periodontal Diseases, and Chapter 6 the Basic Erosive Wear Examination (BEWE). Clear and concise information is provided throughout the book, with relevant learning outcomes listed at the beginning of each chapter.

All health professionals involved in oral health education and promotion are aware that having access to evidence-based information is essential, however in addition to knowledge of the subject, oral health educators must be able to motivate and inspire. This leads to the question, '*Who or what, motivates the motivators?*'

The ability to enthuse and inspire is one of the skills that an oral health educator should have. One cannot fail to recognise the enthusiasm that the authors have for the subject as it is deeply embedded in the script, and that makes this an essential text for those who are delivering oral health education as well as those who aspire to it. The saying, '*enthusiasm cannot be taught as it has to be caught,*' is very relevant to oral health education and promotion, and readers will not only gain the knowledge they need to be effective educators, but also the inspiration and enthusiasm to deliver it.

Rosemarie Khan OBE
OBE, M.Ed., BA, Dip. DH, Dip. DHE, FAETC

Preface

Oral health is central to our general wellbeing. The health of the body begins with the oral cavity, since all our daily nutrients, beneficial or otherwise, pass through it.

Knowledge in the field of oral health changes rapidly, with developments in scientific research, products and technology, and policy. Patients therefore need trained oral health educators (OHEs) and promoters who have the latest knowledge in the field to help prevent and control dental conditions and diseases. It is also vital that dental care professionals (DCPs) and health professionals consistently promote the same messages to avoid confusion, and ultimately improve and maintain oral health within the population.

This book covers the theoretical and practical aspects of oral health education and promotion and is the course companion for UK dental nurses studying oral health education. It is also aimed at dental hygienists, therapists, and dentists who regularly promote and practise oral health education and require up-to-date, evidence-based knowledge. Other professionals, such as health visitors, nurses, dieticians, midwives, and teachers will also find the book invaluable.

Each chapter deals with various aspects of oral health in logical order, and includes *learning outcomes*, detailing what the reader (particularly students) should have learned by the end of each chapter.

After reading this book, the reader should be able to:

- Confidently educate patients about diseases and conditions that affect the oral cavity; their prevention, treatment, and management.
- Plan and undertake a lesson on an oral health topic to an individual and a group.
- Provide a very brief intervention on smoking and alcohol, and signpost patients towards specialist support.
- Give basic advice on diet, nutrition, and exercise.
- Set up a preventive dental unit and an exhibition on an oral health topic.
- Be aware of the wider context of oral and health education and promotion in society.
- Use knowledge gained to help pass a qualification in oral health education.

Acknowledgements

The authors wish to thank Elizabeth Hill, RDN, Cert. OHE (NEBDN) for her expert advice and contributions throughout the book;

Rosemarie Khan, OBE, M.Ed., BA, Dip. DH, Dip. DHE, FAETC (Dental Hygiene Tutor, School for Dental Care Professionals, University Dental Hospital of Manchester) for writing the foreword.

Elizabeth Clark and Stephen MacDonald (of the British Dental Association) for their support.

They are also indebted to the following for imagery:

Dr Ian Bellamy (Principal dentist and practice owner, Aquae Sulis);

British Society of Periodontology;

Paul Chapman for the front cover;

Dr Nick Claydon (Clinical Research Fellow, Clinical Trials Unit, Bristol University);

Carole Hollins (Author and General Dental Practitioner);

Dr Susan Hooper (Honorary Senior Teaching Fellow, Bristol University);

Professor M.A.O. Lewis (Professor of Oral Medicine and Director of Recruitment and Admissions, Cardiff University);

Ruth Macintosh;

Mary Mowbray (RDH) (Chief Executive of the Institute of Dental Hygiene, New Zealand; practice owner Dental Hygiene Clinic, Auckland);

Dr Rachel Sammons (Institute of Clinical Sciences, College of Medical & Dental Sciences, The University of Birmingham);

Elaine Tilling MSc, RDH, DMMS, MIPHE, (TePe Oral Hygiene Products Ltd.);

Professor Nicola West (Professor in Restorative Dentistry, Bristol University).

Acknowledgments

About the Companion Website

Don't forget to visit the companion website for this book:

www.wiley.com/go/felton/oralhealth

There you will find valuable material designed to enhance your learning, including multiple choice questions.

Scan this QR code to visit the companion website

Section 1

Structure and Functions of the Oral Cavity

INTRODUCTION

Part 1 of this book contains one chapter, which looks at the structure and functions of the oral cavity in some detail.

It explores the development of the oral cavity *in utero*, including cleft lip and palate, the structure of the tooth and its supporting tissues, plus eruption dates for primary and secondary dentitions.

It also includes the functions of the tongue in maintaining oral health and common conditions associated with it, plus the composition and role of saliva in keeping the mouth healthy.

Chapter 1

The oral cavity in health

Learning outcomes

By the end of this chapter you should be able to:

1. Describe how the oral cavity, jaws, and face develop *in utero*.
2. Explain the structures and functions of the tissues and fluid of the oral cavity, including teeth, supporting structures, the tongue, and saliva.
3. Distinguish between the different types of cleft lip and cleft palate.
4. List primary and secondary dentition eruption dates.

INTRODUCTION

Before oral health educators (OHEs) can deliver dental health messages to patients and confidently discuss oral care and disease with them, they will need a basic understanding of how the mouth develops *in utero* (in the uterus), the anatomy of the oral cavity (Figures 1.1, 1.2, 1.3, and 1.4), and how the following structures function within it:

- Teeth (including dentition).
- Periodontium (the supporting structure of the tooth).
- Tongue.
- Salivary glands (and saliva).

Basic Guide to Oral Health Education and Promotion, Third Edition.
Alison Chapman and Simon H. Felton.
© 2021 John Wiley & Sons Ltd. Published 2021 by John Wiley & Sons Ltd.
Companion website: www.wiley.com/go/felton/oralhealth

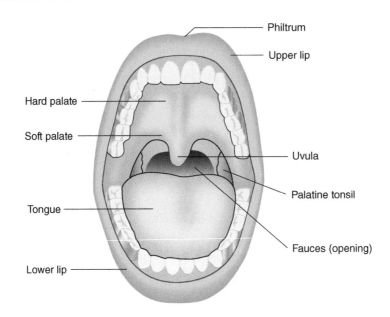

Figure 1.1 Structure of the oral cavity. Source: From [1]. Reproduced with permission of Elsevier.

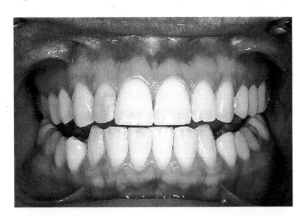

Figure 1.2 A healthy mouth (white person). Source: [2]. Reproduced with permission of Blackwell.

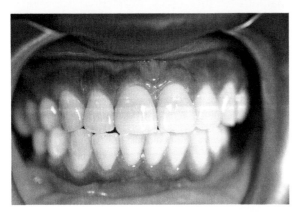

Figure 1.3 A healthy mouth (black person). Source: Alison Chapman.

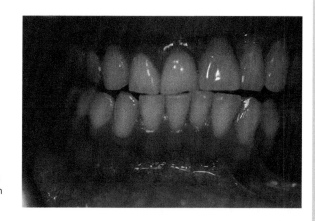

Figure 1.4 A healthy mouth (Asian person). Source: Alison Chapman.

ORAL EMBRYOLOGY

A basic understanding of the development of the face, oral cavity, and jaws in the embryo and developing foetus will help enable the OHE to discuss with patients certain oral manifestations of conditions that stem from *in utero* development; notably cleft lip and palate.

An *embryo* describes the growing organism up to 8 weeks *in utero*; a *foetus* describes the growing organism from 8 weeks *in utero*.

Development of the face

At approximately week 4 *in utero* (Figure 1.5), the embryo begins to develop five facial processes (or projections), which eventually form the face, oral cavity, palate, and jaws by week 8 [3]:

- Frontonasal process – forms the forehead, nose, and philtrum (groove in upper lip).
- Maxillary process (two projections) – forms the middle face and upper lip.
- Mandibular process (two projections) – forms the mandible (lower jaw) and lower lip.

Figure 1.5 Facial development at 4 weeks *in utero*. Source: From [3]. Reproduced with permission of Wiley-Blackwell.

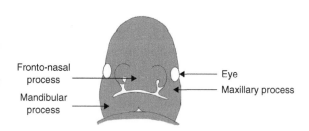

Development of the palate and nasal cavities

Week 5

The frontonasal and maxillary processes begin to form the nose and maxilla (upper jaw). However, if the nasal and maxillary processes fail to fuse, then a cleft will result. This is the most common craniofacial (skull and face) abnormality that babies are born with, and is thought to commonly result from a combination of genetic and environmental factors, or as part of a wider syndrome [4].

A baby can be born with a cleft lip, a cleft palate, or both. Cleft lip and/or palate occurs in 1–2 births out of every 1000 in developed countries [5]. Submucous cleft palate can also occur, which is a cleft in the soft palate and includes a split in the uvula. Surgery to close a gap is often undertaken when a baby is less than a year old.

A cleft lip can be anything from a small notch in the lip (incomplete cleft lip) to a wide gap that runs up to the nostril (complete cleft lip). It can also affect the gum, which, again, can be a small notch or complete separation of the gum.

A cleft lip can be either (Figure 1.6):

- Unilateral – affects one side of the mouth (incomplete or complete).
- Bilateral – affects both sides of the mouth (incomplete or complete).

A cleft palate is a gap in the roof of the mouth. A cleft can affect the soft palate (towards the throat) or the hard palate (towards the lips), or both. Like a cleft lip, a cleft palate can be unilateral or bilateral, and complete or incomplete (Figure 1.6)

Week 6

By week 6, the primary palate and nasal septum have developed. The septum divides the nasal cavity into two.

Week 8

By week 8, the palate is divided into oral and nasal cavities.

Development of the jaws (mandible and maxilla)

Week 6

By week 6, a band of dense fibrous tissue (Meckel's cartilage) forms and provides the structure around which the mandible forms.

Week 7

By week 7, bone develops, outlining the body of the mandible.

As the bone grows backwards two secondary cartilages develop; these eventually become the condyle and coronoid processes.

As the bone grows forward, the two sides are separated by a cartilage called the mandibular symphysis. The two sides will finally fuse into one bone approximately 2 years after birth.

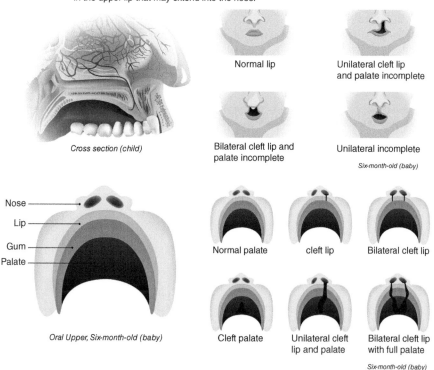

Pediatric
Cleft Lip and Palate

Cleft lip and cleft palate, also known as orofacial cleft, is a group of conditions that includes cleft lip (CL), cleft palate (CP). A cleft lip contains an opening in the upper lip that may extend into the nose.

Cross section (child)

Normal lip

Unilateral cleft lip and palate incomplete

Bilateral cleft lip and palate incomplete

Unilateral incomplete

Six-month-old (baby)

Nose
Lip
Gum
Palate

Oral Upper, Six-month-old (baby)

Normal palate

cleft lip

Bilateral cleft lip

Cleft palate

Unilateral cleft lip and palate

Bilateral cleft lip with full palate

Six-month-old (baby)

Figure 1.6 Cleft lip and palate in a six-month-old baby. Source: Dreamstime.com/Pattarawit Chompipat | ID 84347343. Reproduced with permission of Dreamstime.com.

Upward growth of bone begins along the mandibular arch forming the alveolar process, which will go on to surround the developing tooth germs.

Week 8
By week 8, ossification (bone development) of the maxilla begins.

Tooth germ development in the foetus

Tooth germ (tissue mass) develops in three stages known as bud, cap, and bell. The developing tooth germ can be affected by the mother's health (see Chapter 20).

1. Bud – at 8 weeks, clumps of cells form swellings called enamel organs. Each enamel organ is responsible for the development of a tooth.

2. Cap – the enamel organ continues to grow and by 12 weeks (the late cap stage), cells have formed the inner enamel epithelium and the outer enamel epithelium. Beneath the inner enamel epithelium, the concentration of cells will eventually become the pulp. The enamel organ is surrounded by a fibrous capsule (the dental follicle), which will eventually form the periodontal ligament.
3. Bell – by 14 weeks, the enamel organ will comprise different layers, which will continue to develop to form the various parts of the tooth.

MAIN FUNCTIONS OF THE ORAL CAVITY

The oral cavity is uniquely designed to carry out two main functions:

1. Begin the process of digestion. The cavity's hard and soft tissues, lubricated by saliva, are designed to withstand the stresses of:
   * Biting.
   * Chewing.
   * Swallowing.
2. Produce speech.

TEETH

Different types of teeth are designed (shaped) to carry out different functions. For example, canines are sharp and pointed for gripping and tearing food, while molars have flatter surfaces for chewing. Tooth form in relation to function is called morphology.

Dental nurses and healthcare workers may remember from their elementary studies that there are two types of dentition (a term used to describe the type, number and arrangement of natural teeth):

1. Primary (deciduous) dentition – consisting of 20 baby teeth.
2. Secondary (permanent) dentition – consisting of 32 adult teeth.

Primary dentition

There are three types of deciduous teeth that make up the primary dentition (Figure 1.7): incisors, canines, and molars (first and second). Table 1.1 details their notation (the code used by the dental profession to identify teeth), approximate eruption dates, and functions.

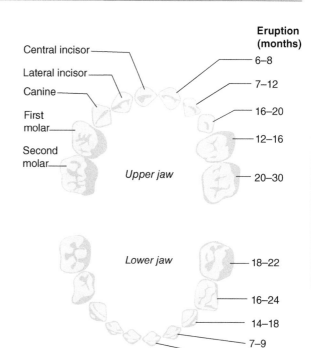

Eruption (months)

Central incisor — 6–8

Lateral incisor — 7–12

Canine — 16–20

First molar — 12–16

Second molar —

Upper jaw — 20–30

Lower jaw — 18–22

— 16–24

— 14–18

— 7–9

— 6–8

Primary dentition

Figure 1.7 Primary dentition. Source: From [1]. Reproduced with permission of Elsevier.

Table 1.1 Primary dentition (notation, approximate eruption dates, and functions).

Tooth	Notation	Approximate eruption date	Function
Incisors	(a & b)	6–12 months (usually lowers first)	Biting
First molars	(d)	12–24 months	Chewing
Canines	(c)	14–20 months	Tearing
Second molars	(e)	18–30 months	Chewing

Table 1.2 FDI World Dental Federation notation for deciduous (primary) dentition.

Patient's upper right (5)	Patient's upper left (6)
55 54 53 52 51	61 62 63 64 65
85 84 83 82 81	71 72 73 74 75
Patient's lower right (8)	Patient's lower left (7)

Table 1.2 details the FDI World Dental Federation notation for primary dentition, which is a charting system commonly used by dentists to associate information to a specific tooth; where the quadrant number is the first digit applied, and the second number identifies the individual tooth.

Secondary dentition

There are four types of permanent teeth that make up the secondary dentition (Figure 1.8): incisors, canines, premolars, and molars. Table 1.3 details their notation, approximate exfoliation/eruption dates, and functions. Table 1.4 details the FDI World Dental Federation notation for secondary dentition.

It is important to remember that these exfoliation/eruption dates are only approximate and vary considerably in children and adolescents. The educator should be prepared to answer questions from parents who are worried that their child's teeth are not erupting at the same age as their friends' teeth. Parents often do not realise, for example, that no teeth fall out to make room for the first permanent molars (sixes), which appear behind the deciduous molars.

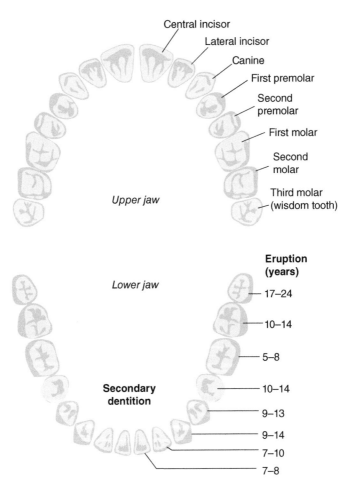

Figure 1.8 Secondary dentition. Source: From [1]. Reproduced with permission of Elsevier.

Table 1.3 Secondary dentition (notation, approximate exfoliation/eruption dates, and functions).

Tooth	Notation	Approximate exfoliation/ eruption dates	Function
First molars	(6)	6–7 years	Chewing
Lower central incisors	(1)	6–7 years	Biting
Upper central incisors	(1)	6–7 years	Biting
Lower lateral incisors	(2)	7–8 years	Biting
Upper lateral incisors	(2)	7–8 years	Biting
Lower canines	(3)	9–10 years	Tearing
First premolars	(4)	10–11 years	Chewing
Second premolars	(5)	11–12 years	Chewing
Upper canines	(3)	11–12 years	Tearing
Second molars	(7)	12–13 years	Chewing
Third molars	(8)	17–24 years	Chewing

Table 1.4 FDI World Dental Federation notation for permanent (secondary) dentition.

Patient's upper right (1)	Patient's upper left (2)
18 17 16 15 14 13 12 11	21 22 23 24 25 26 27 28
48 47 46 45 44 43 42 41	31 32 33 34 35 36 37 38
Patient's lower right (4)	Patient's lower left (3)

Structure of the tooth

Tooth structure (Figure 1.9) is complex and comprises several different hard layers that protect a soft, inner pulp (nerves and blood vessels).

Organic and inorganic tooth matter

The terms *organic* and *inorganic* are often mentioned in connection with tooth structure. Educators must know what these terms mean and their percentages in hard tooth structures.

Organic means *living* and describes the matrix (framework) of water, cells, fibres and proteins, which make the tooth a living structure.

Inorganic means *non-living* and describes the mineral content of the tooth, which gives it its strength. These minerals are complex calcium salts.

Table 1.5 shows the percentages of organic and inorganic matter in hard tooth structures.

It is also important to know the basic details about these three hard tooth substances, and also pulp.

Enamel

Enamel (Figure 1.9) is made up of prisms (crystals of hydroxyapatite) arranged vertically in a wavy pattern, which give it great strength. The prisms, which

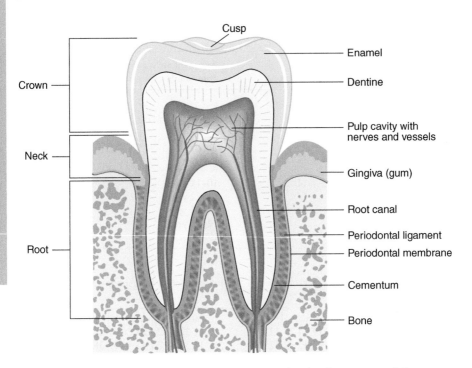

Figure 1.9 Structure of the tooth. Source: From [1]. Reproduced with permission of Elsevier.

Table 1.5   Percentages of organic and inorganic matter in hard tooth structures.

Structure	Inorganic	Organic
Enamel	96%	4%
Dentine	70%	30%
Cementum	45%	55%

resemble fish scales, are supported by a matrix of organic material including keratinised (*horn-like*) cells, which can be seen under an electron microscope.

Properties of enamel
Enamel is:

- The hardest substance in the human body.
- Brittle – it fractures when the underlying dentine is weakened by decay (caries).
- Insensitive to stimuli (e.g. hot, cold, and sweet substances).
- Darkens slightly with age – as secondary dentine is laid down and stains from proteins in the diet, tannin-rich food and drinks, and smoking are absorbed.

Enamel is also subject to three types of wear and tear (see Chapter 6). The educator needs to be aware of these and able to differentiate between them:

1. Erosion – usually seen on palatal and lingual (next to palate and tongue) surfaces.
2. Abrasion – usually seen on cervical (outer neck of tooth) surfaces.
3. Attrition – natural wear often seen on occlusal (biting) surfaces.

Dentine

Dentine constitutes the main bulk of the tooth (Figure 1.9) and consists of millions of microscopic tubules (fine tubes), running in a curved pattern from the pulp to the enamel on the crown and the cementum on the root.

Properties of dentine

Dentine is:

- Softer than enamel, but harder than cementum and bone.
- Light yellow in colour.
- Sensitive to stimuli (e.g. hot, cold, and sweet substances). Reasons for this sensitivity are not fully understood, but it usually lessens with age.

Dentine also changes throughout life. After a tooth is fully developed, more dentine is laid down and is called secondary dentine.

Cementum

Cementum covers the surface of the root (Figure 1.9) and provides an attachment for the periodontal ligament. The fibres of the ligament are fixed in the cementum and in the alveolar bone (see supporting structures of the tooth).

Properties of cementum

Cementum is of similar hardness to bone and thickens throughout life to counteract wear and tear caused by chewing and movement.

Pulp

Pulp is a soft living tissue within the pulp chamber and root canal of the tooth (Figure 1.9). It consists of blood vessels, nerves, fibres, and cells.

Properties of pulp

The pulp chamber shrinks with age as more secondary dentine is laid down, so that the tooth becomes less vulnerable to damage.

Supporting structures of the tooth

The periodontium (Figure 1.10) is the collective name for the supporting structures of the tooth.

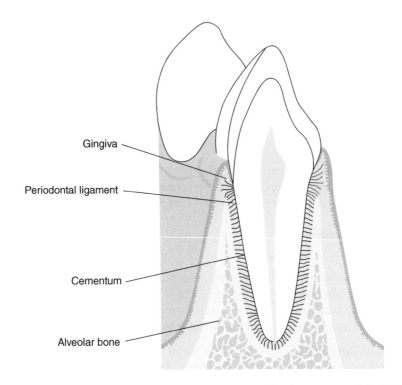

Gingiva

Periodontal ligament

Cementum

Alveolar bone

Figure 1.10 The periodontium. Source: From [6]. Reproduced with permission of Blackwell.

It comprises:

- Periodontal ligament.
- Cementum (part of the tooth and supporting structure).
- Alveolar bone (see later in chapter). This develops as the tooth erupts, forming the alveolus of the mandible and maxilla.
- Gingivae (gums).

The periodontal ligament

The periodontal ligament is a connective tissue that holds the tooth in place in the alveolar bone (assisted by cementum). The ligament is between 0.1–0.3 mm wide and contains blood vessels, nerves, cells, and collagen fibres [7].

The collagen fibres attach the tooth to the alveolar bone and run in different directions, which provide strength and flexibility, and act as a shock absorber for the tooth; teeth need to move slightly in their sockets in order to withstand the pressures of mastication (chewing). Imagine what it would feel like to bite hard with teeth rigidly cemented into bone.

Cementum

See *Structure of the tooth*.

Alveolar bone (also known as the alveolar ridge)

Alveolar bones are horseshoe-shaped projections of the maxilla and mandible. They provide an attachment for the fibres of the periodontal ligament, sockets for the teeth, and support the teeth by absorbing and distributing occlusal forces.

Gingivae

The gingivae (gums) consist of mucous membranes and underlying fibrous tissue, covering the alveolar bone.

Gingivae are divided into four sections (Figure 1.11):

1. Attached gingiva – a firm, pale pink (but may have some brown pigmentation), stippled gum tightly attached to the underlying alveolar bone. It is keratinised (hard and firm-like horn) to withstand the friction of chewing. Its orange-peel appearance (stippling) comes from tightly packed bundles of collagen fibres that attach it to the bone. Loss of stippling is one of the signs of gingivitis (see Chapter 3).
2. Free gingiva – where the gum meets the tooth. It is less tightly attached and not stippled. It is also keratinised and contoured to form little points of gum between teeth – the interdental papillae. The indentation between attached and free gingiva is called the free gingival groove.

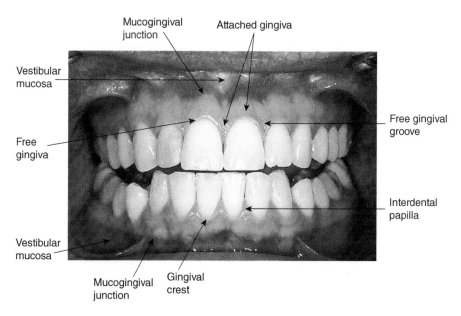

Figure 1.11 Gingivae. Source: [2]. Reproduced with permission of Blackwell.

3. Gingival crest – the edge of the gum and interdental papillae bordering the tooth. Behind the crest is the gingival sulcus (or crevice), which is not more than 2 mm in depth [7]. This base of the crevice is lined with a layer of cells called the junctional epithelium, which attaches the gum to the tooth. When this epithelium breaks down, in disease, periodontal ligament fibres are exposed to bacterial enzymes and toxins. As these fibres break down, a periodontal pocket is formed.
4. Mucogingival junction – the meeting point of the keratinised attached gingiva and the non-keratinised vestibular mucosa (soft, dark red tissue, which lines the inside of lips, cheeks, and the floor of the mouth).

THE TONGUE AND THE FLOOR OF THE MOUTH

The tongue is a muscular, mobile organ, which lies in the floor of the mouth, and is comprised of four surfaces:

1. Dorsal (upper) surface – covered by a thick, keratinised epithelium to withstand chewing, and a large number of projections called papillae. These papillae contain taste buds. The dorsal surface is divided into two sections:
   * Anterior (front) two-thirds (against the palate).
   * Posterior (back) third (towards the pharynx).
2. Ventral (under) surface – covered by a thin mucous membrane. In the middle of the front section, the mucosa is divided by a sharp fold (the *lingual frenulum*), which joins the tip of the tongue to the floor of the mouth.
3. Tip – the pointed front, which can be protruded or moved around the mouth by muscular action. For a baby, the tip of the tongue is an important sensory organ, which explores and identifies objects. It also acts as a great natural cleanser, removing food debris.
4. Root – the deep attachment of the tongue, which forms the anterior surface of the pharynx.

Muscles of the tongue

There are two groups of tongue muscles:

1. Intrinsic (inside) – which can alter its shape.
2. Extrinsic (outside) – which move the tongue and also help alter its shape.

Functions of the tongue

The main functions of the tongue are:

* Taste.
* Mastication (chewing).

- Deglutition (swallowing).
- Speech.
- Cleansing.
- Protection.

Taste

The tongue (and other parts of the oral cavity) is covered with taste buds that allow us to distinguish between sweet, sour, salt, bitter, and umami (savoury) tastes. An adult has approximately 9000 taste buds, which are mainly situated on the upper surface of the tongue (there are also some on the palate and even on the throat) [7].

Mastication

The tongue helps pass a soft mass of chewed food (bolus) along its dorsal surface and presses it against the hard palate.

Deglutition

The tongue helps pass the bolus towards the entrance of the oesophagus.

Speech

Tongue movement plays a major part in the production of different sounds.

Natural cleansing

Tongue muscles allow for tremendous movement, and the tongue can help remove food particles from all areas of the mouth (mainly using the tip).

Protection

The tongue moves saliva (which has an antibacterial property) around the oral cavity.

Conditions affecting the tongue

The following conditions affect the tongue (see Chapter 8 for more detail/images):

- Glossitis (inflammation of the tongue) – a symptom of conditions such as dry mouth, infections, injury from a burn, irritants, vitamin B complex deficiency, skin conditions (e.g. lichen planus), or an allergic reaction. The underlying cause needs to be treated.
- Soreness of the tongue, which may be due to a variety of reasons, including anaemia, vitamin B complex deficiency, and hormonal imbalance.
- Black hairy tongue – due to overgrowth of tongue papillae, stained by chromogenic bacteria, mouthwash (e.g. chlorhexidine gluconate), or smoking. Looks alarming, but is not serious.

- Geographic tongue (also called benign migratory glossitis) – smooth map-like irregular areas on the dorsal surface (where the papillae are missing), which come and go. It can be harmless, but is sometimes sore and often runs in families. It can also be an indication of other systemic conditions [7].

Piercing of the tongue can also cause problems and the educator should be able to advise patients on this matter (see Chapter 22).

The floor of the mouth

The educator must know that the floor of the mouth consists of a muscle called the mylohyoid and associated structures.

SALIVA

Incredible stuff, saliva! It is often taken for granted, and patients only realise how vital it is to the wellbeing of the oral cavity and the whole body, when its flow is diminished (see Chapter 7). Saliva is secreted by three major and numerous minor salivary glands. The minor glands are found in the lining of the oral cavity, on the inside of the lips, the cheeks, the palate, and even the pharynx.

Major salivary glands

The three major salivary glands (Figure 1.12) are as follows:

1. Parotid gland – situated in front of the ear. It is the largest salivary gland and produces 25% of the total volume of saliva [7]. It makes serous (watery) saliva, which is transported into the oral cavity by the parotid duct that opens adjacent to the upper molars. The parotid gland swells during mumps (*parotitis*).
2. Submandibular gland – situated beneath the mylohyoid muscle towards the base of the mandible. It is the middle of the three glands, in both size and position, and produces a mixture of serous and mucous saliva. It accounts for around 70% of total saliva and opens via the submandibular duct on the floor of the mouth [7].

   When dental nurses assist the dentist, they may occasionally notice a small fountain as the saliva appears from this duct (which can also happen when yawning).

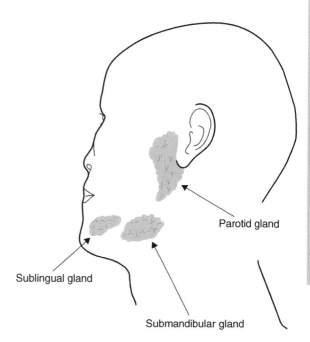

Figure 1.12 Major salivary glands. Source: From [8]. Reproduced with permission of Blackwell.

Parotid gland

Sublingual gland

Submandibular gland

3. Sublingual gland – is also situated beneath the anterior floor of the mouth under the front of the tongue. It produces 5% of total saliva [7], mainly in the form of mucous, which drains through numerous small ducts on the ridge of the sublingual fold (the area next to the frenulum beneath the anterior of tongue).

Composition of saliva

Saliva is made up of 99.5% water and 0.5% dissolved substances, although the composition varies between individuals [7].

Dissolved substances include:

- Mucins – these are glycoproteins that give saliva its viscosity (stickiness), lubricate the oral tissues, and are the origin of the salivary pellicle (the sticky film which forms on teeth within minutes of cleaning).
- Enzymes – there are many, but the OHE needs only to remember the main ones:
  - Salivary amylase (ptyalin), which converts starch into maltose.
  - Lysozyme, which attacks the cell walls of bacteria, thus protecting the oral cavity from invading pathogens.
- Serum proteins – albumin and globulin (saliva is formed from serum; the watery basis of blood).

- Waste products – urea and uric acid.
- Gases – oxygen, nitrogen, and carbon dioxide in solution. The latter vaporises when it enters the mouth and is given off as a gas.
- Inorganic ions – including sodium, sulphate, potassium, calcium, phosphate, and chloride. The important ones to remember are calcium and phosphate ions, which are concerned with remineralisation of the teeth after an acid attack (see Chapter 5) and the development of calculus (see Chapter 2).
- Saliva also contains large numbers of microorganisms and remnants of food substances.

Functions of saliva

There are eight main functions of saliva:

1. Aids mastication and deglutition – mucous helps form the food bolus.
2. Oral hygiene – washing and antibacterial action helps control disease of the oral cavity. Lysozyme controls bacterial growth. This is why saliva is said to have antibacterial properties, and why animals instinctively lick their wounds.
3. Speech – a lubricant. For example, nervousness = production of adrenaline = reduction in saliva = dry mouth.
4. Taste – saliva dissolves substances and allows the taste buds to recognise taste.
5. Helps maintain water balance (of body) – when water balance is low, saliva is reduced, producing thirst.
6. Excretion – trace amounts of urea and uric acid (a minor role in total body excretion).
7. Digestion – salivary amylase begins the breakdown of cooked starch (a relatively minor role in the whole digestive process, but important in relation to sucrose intake and oral disease).
8. Buffering action – helps maintain the neutral pH of the mouth. The bicarbonate ion is vital to the health of the mouth as it is concerned with the buffering action of saliva. The average resting pH of the mouth (when no food has just been consumed) is 6.7. This is neutral, neither acid nor alkaline. (pH is a symbol used to indicate measurement of acidity or alkalinity of substances or liquids, and stands for the German term *potenz Hydrogen*.)

Facts about saliva

Here are some general points of interest about saliva:

- More is secreted when required (reflex action).
- Composition varies according to what is being eaten (e.g. more mucous with meat).

- Average amount produced daily by adults is 0.5–1 L. Certain medical conditions and disabilities cause the overproduction of saliva, resulting in dribbling (e.g. patients with Down's syndrome and Parkinson's disease, and fungal infections, such as angular cheilitis – see Chapter 8).
- Flow almost ceases during sleep.
- Saliva is sterile until it enters the mouth.
- Saliva tests can be used to solve crimes, since saliva contains deoxyribonucleic acid (DNA), which can be used to help identify individuals. Dental companies sell saliva testing kits, which can be used by OHEs to demonstrate saliva pH to patients.

Other additives within the mouth

Although saliva entering the mouth is sterile, it soon loses this property as it collects organic materials that are already present, including:

- Microorganisms: bacteria (mainly *streptococci*), viruses (e.g. herpes simplex), and fungi (e.g. *Candida albicans*).
- Leucocytes (white blood cells), which fight infection. Not present in *edentulous* (toothless) babies or in saliva collected from the duct, so presumed to come from gingival crevice after teeth erupt.
- Dietary substances (meal remains).

REFERENCES

1. Thibodeau, G.A. & Patton, K.T. (2002) *Anatomy and Physiology*. 5th edn. Mosby, Missouri.
2. Lang, N.P., Mombelli, A. & Attström, R. (2003) Dental plaque and calculus. In: *Clinical Periodontology and Implant Dentistry* (eds. J. Lindhe, T. Karring & N.P. Lang N.P.), 4th edn, pp. 81–105. Blackwell Munksgaard, Oxford.
3. Phillips, S. Oral embryology, histology and anatomy. In: *Clinical Textbook of Dental Hygiene and Therapy* (ed. S.L Noble), 2nd edn. pp. 3–5. Wiley-Blackwell, Oxford.
4. Cleft Lip & Palate Association. (2019). *What is Cleft Lip & Palate?* Available at: https://www.clapa.com/what-is-cleft-lip-palate/ [accessed 13 March 2019].
5. Watkins, S.E., Meyer, R.E., Strauss, R.P., Aylsworth, A.S. (2014) Classification, epidemiology, and genetics of orofacial clefts. *Clinics in Plastic Surgery*, 41(2), 149–163.
6. Lindhe, J., Karring, T. & Araújo, M. Anatomy of the periodontium. In: *Clinical Periodontology and Implant Dentistry* (eds. J.T. Lindhe, T. Karring & N.P. Lang). 4th edn, pp. 3–49. Blackwell Munksgaard, Oxford.
7. Collins, W.J., Walsh, T. & Figures, K. (1999) *A Handbook for Dental Hygienists*. 4th edn. Butterworth Heinemann, Oxford.
8. Fejerskov, O. & Kidd, E. (2003) *Dental Caries: The Disease and its Clinical Management*. Blackwell Munksgaard, Oxford.

Section 2

Diseases and Conditions of the Oral Cavity

INTRODUCTION

This section explores the reasons for, and the effects of, the breakdown of oral health, and details advice that should be given to patients to control disease and restore a good standard of oral health.

What causes oral disease?

There is, of course, no brief answer. The determinants are many and complex, and more often than not a combination of factors is involved in the development of a particular condition or disease: genetic, cultural, environmental, socioeconomic, diet, and lifestyle.

Education is vital in controlling dental disease, and that is where the oral health educator (OHE) can help.

Chapter 2

Plaque, calculus, and staining

Learning outcomes

By the end of this chapter you should be able to:

1. Explain the causes and development of plaque, and advise on plaque control.
2. Distinguish between *aerobic* and *anaerobic* bacteria and their effects on oral tissues.
3. List secondary factors in the development of plaque.
4. Explain the types, causes and effects of calculus, and its treatment.
5. Differentiate between *intrinsic* and *extrinsic* tooth staining, their causes and treatment (including whitening).

INTRODUCTION

Oral health educators (OHEs) need an understanding of plaque and calculus, and their roles in the development of common dental diseases, such as caries, gingivitis, and periodontitis. The OHE should also be able to distinguish between intrinsic and extrinsic staining, and answer patient questions on teeth whitening.

PLAQUE

Most people have heard of plaque, but few would be able to explain its composition.

Basic Guide to Oral Health Education and Promotion, Third Edition.
Alison Chapman and Simon H. Felton.
© 2021 John Wiley & Sons Ltd. Published 2021 by John Wiley & Sons Ltd.
Companion website: www.wiley.com/go/felton/oralhealth

Plaque is a soft, non-calcified adherent film that collects on the surfaces of teeth, and comprises approximately:

- 70% microorganisms (bacteria, fungi, viruses).
- 30% matrix (the framework that holds it together).

Plaque is found in all mouths and makes up part of the natural flora of the body. The most common sites where plaque is found are occlusal pits and fissures, cervical margins of the teeth and in periodontal pockets. Patients can be made aware of plaque in their mouths by using a disclosing solution or tablets (Figure 2.1 a,b). (See Chapter 19.)

Plaque is a major causative factor in gingival and periodontal disease and a contributory factor in dental caries. Even in people with good toothbrushing

(a)

(b)

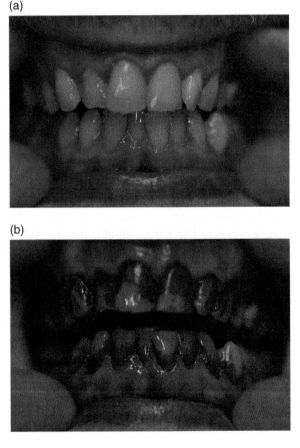

Figure 2.1 (a,b) Plaque undisclosed (a) disclosed (b) in the same mouth. Source: Alison Chapman.

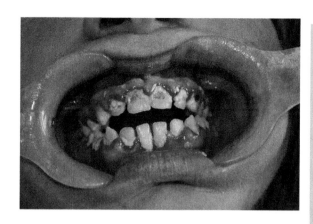

Figure 2.2 Mature plaque and gingivitis in a neglected mouth. Source: Alison Chapman.

skills, one would need to brush and floss approximately every 3 minutes in order to prevent plaque from forming.

In a healthy mouth, there is a natural balance of bacteria, but when illness or antibiotics (for example) upset the balance of the mouth's flora, or when teeth are not cleaned often and/or appropriately, plaque matures. Waste products from the bacteria, enzymes and toxins then cause an inflammatory response in the gingival tissues leading to gingivitis (Figure 2.2). Depending on an individual's response, gingivitis can progress to periodontal disease.

Biofilms

Dental plaque is a type of biofilm, and the concept of a biofilm is of huge importance not only to dentistry, but also to the wider medical world and many sectors of industry. Since the 1990s, there has been a huge amount of research into biofilms, which reflects our growing understanding of their importance.

A biofilm, in simple terms, is a thin layer of bacteria that adheres to a surface. Over 95% of bacteria in nature exist in a biofilm state as opposed to living independently, and over 500 species of bacteria have been identified in oral plaque biofilms. Contact lenses, rocks in rivers and aspirator tubing in the dental surgery are all examples of surfaces colonised by biofilms.

Within a biofilm, bacteria are not just sitting alongside one another passively; they are communicating, interacting, and gaining benefits from one another – acting as a team. This is what makes a biofilm so virulent, resilient, and difficult to manage.

Bacteria

Bacteria is the most common microorganism found in the plaque biofilm, and can be classified as to whether they need oxygen (aerobic) or not (anaerobic) to survive.

Aerobic bacteria

The majority of bacteria in a healthy mouth come from the oxygen-dependent (aerobic) *streptococci* genus, which colonise areas of the mouth where oxygen is readily available. When resistance is lowered, they can give rise to sore throats and other illnesses, but are generally less potentially harmful than their non-oxygen-dependent (anaerobic) relatives.

The most common species of streptococci bacteria found in the oral cavity are:

- *Streptococcus sanguis.*
- *Streptococcus mutans.*
- *Streptococcus mitis.*
- *Streptococcus salivarius.*

Aerobic bacteria feed on sucrose from the human diet and produce sticky substances that enable other more harmful organisms to attach themselves, causing plaque to become more dense and harmful to tissues.

Anaerobic bacteria

Anaerobic bacteria are a more potentially *pathogenic* (disease causing) bacteria, when displaced from their normal habitat. They produce enzymes and toxins and do not need oxygen to survive. They can be found in deeper layers of plaque and in areas of the mouth, such as periodontal pockets, which render them difficult to remove. Examples of anaerobic bacteria are:

- Fusiforms.
- Vibrios.
- Spirochaetes.

Other microorganisms found in plaque

As well as bacteria, other microorganisms found in plaque, include fungi and viruses.

Fungi

Fungi, such as *Candida albicans,* are also commonly found in plaque. As with bacteria, these do not affect oral health unless the body's resistance is lowered and the immune system is upset, in which case they can cause dental thrush or stomatitis (see Chapter 8).

Viruses

The most common virus in the oral cavity is herpes simplex, which gives rise to cold sores (see Chapter 8).

The matrix

In addition to providing an abundant food source for bacteria, plaque also collects other debris present in the mouth, which forms the *matrix* (in which the colonising bacteria feed and reproduce).

The following substances make up the matrix:

- Proteins and carbohydrates (from food debris).
- Dead cells (from oral tissues).
- Red blood cells.
- White blood cells.
- Antigens (involved in the body's immune response).
- Enzymes and toxins (produced by bacteria).
- Lactic acid.
- Mineral salts.

Stages in plaque formation

Stage 1

Saliva plays a large part in the formation of plaque, and within a few minutes of cleaning, the tooth is covered in a sticky film made from salivary proteins, called the salivary pellicle. This provides receptors for early bacterial colonisers to attach to. Initially, these connections are weak and easily broken. These early aerobic bacteria are gram-positive (stain violet when exposed to Gram's stain in the laboratory), and feed on sugars from the diet.

Stage 2

Bacteria begin to produce substances that anchor them to the pellicle, thus increasing the adhesive properties of plaque. The matrix builds, with some matrix components made by bacteria themselves.

Stage 3

Bacteria begin to produce carbon dioxide and also excrete waste products. The environment becomes more attractive to gram-negative species (which stain red when exposed to Gram's stain). The plaque becomes thicker and denser as it matures, and contains diverse species that have a potential to cause disease. Mushroom-shaped 'clouds' of matrix form with channels running between them to facilitate the movement of nutrients and waste products (Figure 2.3).

Stage 4

As the biofilm thickens, some bacteria start to die or break off to form new colonies. Bacteria within the colony reproduce to replace those that have broken away or died, and the cycle continues.

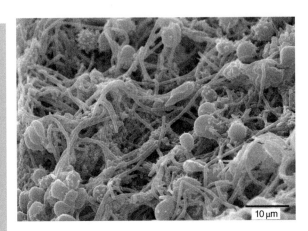

Figure 2.3 Mature plaque (scanning electron microscope). Source: Dr Rachel Sammons. Reproduced with permission of Institute of Clinical Sciences, College of Medical & Dental Sciences, The University of Birmingham.

10 μm

Local risk factors in the retention of plaque

The importance of the following local risk factors in the retention of plaque (and therefore in the development of dental disease) should not be underestimated:

- Large or uneven restorations.
- Bridges.
- Crowns with poor margins.
- Implants.
- Dentures and obturators.
- Orthodontic appliances.
- Calculus.
- Periodontal pockets.

Plaque control

The following measures should be taken to prevent the build-up of plaque:

- Physical (i.e. toothbrushing and interdental cleaning).
- Chemical (e.g. chlorhexidine mouthwashes) – not needed by all patients.
- A low sucrose diet.

Remember! The enzymes and toxins of anaerobic bacteria in mature plaque are the primary causes of gingivitis, which can lead to periodontitis. It is therefore vital that the patient removes plaque in order to prevent the onset of these more serious conditions.

CALCULUS

Calculus is a mineralised hard deposit of calcium salts that forms in plaque. It is found on teeth and other solid structures in the mouth and plays a role in the development of periodontal disease by attracting more plaque.

Patients sometimes refer to calculus (a Latin word meaning *stone*) as *tartar* or *scale*. When talking to patients, it is worth mentioning that these three terms mean the same thing. Some patients get confused between plaque and calculus and think that they are one and the same, and so the differences between them should be explained in simple terms. Other patients know what calculus looks like and complain of its build-up around the lower incisors.

Calculus consists of approximately:

- 70% inorganic salts.
- 30% microorganisms and organic materials.

Types of Calculus

There are two main types of calculus:

1. Supragingival – which forms above the gingival margin.
2. Subgingival – which forms in the periodontal pocket.

Supragingival calculus

Supragingival calculus (Figure 2.4) begins to form after 2–14 days of inadequate plaque removal, depending upon the individual's cleaning ability and mineral content of their saliva. Most supragingival calculus is found on teeth

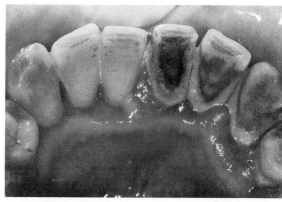

Figure 2.4 Supragingival calculus before (right) and after (left) scaling. Source: Mary Mowbray. Reproduced with permission of Mary Mowbray.

adjacent to the main saliva ducts, i.e. behind the lower central incisors and on the buccal (cheek) surfaces of the upper first and second molars.

Supragingival calculus is usually preceded by plaque accumulation that becomes hardened (calcified) by the mineral salts in saliva (i.e. calcium and phosphate salts become incorporated into sticky plaque, causing calcification).

Some patients have more supragingival calculus than others, and this is because they:

• Have relatively more calcium and phosphate ions in saliva, and/or
• Do not remove plaque effectively, and so there is a material present for saliva to calcify.
• Have highly alkaline saliva, which favours the production of calculus.

Patients cannot remove calculus with a brush or floss once it has hardened, and because it has a rough texture, more plaque adheres, and the process of calcification begins again. Dentists and hygienists scale and polish teeth to remove supragingival calculus (and help prevent periodontal disease).

Subgingival calculus

Subgingival calculus (Figure 2.5) is less obvious to the patient, and is found below the gum margin in periodontal pockets. It is often black, dark brown or green in colour and is formed when minerals from fluid (crevicular fluid) in the gingival crevice come into contact with plaque. (The dark colour is derived from the breakdown of blood constituents resulting from ulceration in the crevice.)

Subgingival calculus is often hard and difficult to remove. Its presence is much more significant than supragingival deposits as it indicates that periodontitis is present.

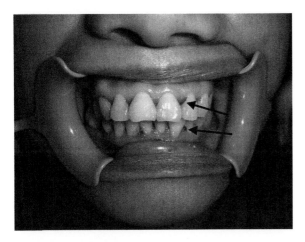

Figure 2.5 Subgingival calculus exposed after improved oral hygiene. Source: Mary Mowbray. Reproduced with permission of Mary Mowbray.

TOOTH STAINING

There are two types of staining that can affect the tooth:

- Intrinsic.
- Extrinsic.

Intrinsic staining

Intrinsic staining occurs within the tooth structure during its development (before birth, or during early childhood), and before it erupts (except in cases of pulpal death, usually caused by trauma). Intrinsic stains cannot be removed, although tooth whitening can conceal them. The whitened tooth will continue to darken with age, but the whitening process can be topped up so that intrinsic stains remain concealed.

Causes of intrinsic staining include:

- Tetracycline – an antibiotic. Taken by a baby or young child, or passed to the foetus by pregnant mother (white, yellow, brown, and grey colours). Not recommended for children under 12 years old or pregnant women.
- Fluoride taken in excess – from tablets, swallowing toothpaste, and naturally occurring high levels in water supply. This is called fluorosis (see Chapter 11).
- Systemic (whole body) upset. Premature birth, acute illness of a baby, young child or pregnant mother can cause hypoplasia – the underdevelopment of a tooth, and therefore enamel (see Chapter 8).
- Rare, inherited imperfections in enamel or dentine – e.g. *amelogenesis imperfecta, dentinogenesis imperfecta* (see Chapter 8).
- Death of pulp. This causes the tooth to progressively darken.
- Age – teeth naturally darken with age.

Extrinsic staining

Extrinsic staining occurs on enamel surfaces after a tooth has erupted, when pigments from the following substances stain the salivary pellicle:

- Tannin (in tea, coffee, and red wine).
- Tobacco (smoking or chewing).
- Betel nut (*paan, gutka,* or *quid*) chewing in certain ethnic groups (Figure 2.6).
- Mouthwash (such as those containing chlorhexidine and essential oils).
- Iron supplements.
- Foods – e.g. berries and turmeric.

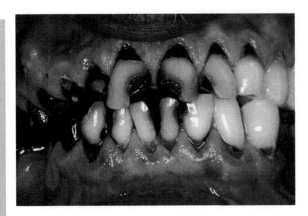

Figure 2.6 Extrinsic staining caused by betel nut chewing. Source: Dr Susan Hooper, Bristol University. Reproduced with permission of Susan Hooper.

Extrinsic stains can be removed with scaling and polishing or by air polishing using a mild abrasive powder.

Occasionally, patients with clean mouths develop a dark stain on lingual and palatal tooth surfaces, which is difficult to remove. This is called *black stain* and the cause is unknown. Children can also develop *green stain*, when the membrane covering an erupting tooth remains and is stained by bacteria. This is usually seen on the buccal surfaces of the upper incisors, can look unsightly, and is often difficult to remove.

Teeth whitening

Although the OHE cannot undertake tooth whitening in the UK, they should be aware of what is involved and its benefits and limitations in case they need to answer a patient's question.

Under the General Dental Council's *Scope of Practice* (see Chapter 31), in the UK only registered dental professionals (dentists, therapists and hygienists) can provide tooth whitening as it is considered a form of dentistry, and should only be undertaken following an assessment by a registered dentist [1]. Therapists and hygienists must have a prescription from the dentist before providing this treatment. Some beauty salons offer teeth whitening, but this is illegal in the UK.

Products that contain or release less than 0.1% hydrogen peroxide can be legally sold in Europe, but unregistered individuals cannot legally use them to provide treatment [1].

Patients should be advised that illegal treatment and home teeth whitening kits can put their oral health at risk, particularly from ill-fitting whitening trays which may cause the gel to leak into the gums and the rest of the oral cavity, and cause sensitivity, or even blistering.

Patients may also ask about toothpaste products, but these often have insufficient whitening product to make a significant difference; they may help remove stains, but will not penetrate the tooth tissue itself.

Teeth whitening in the practice

Teeth whitening carried out in the practice can make a significant difference to the colour of teeth. Whitening does not cause any damage to teeth and can be used for patients over 18 years old. It simply changes the colour of dentine, so it can be used for patients affected by systemic intrinsic staining, such as tetracycline, as well as extrinsic stains caused by tea, coffee, tobacco products, and red wine.

The process uses gels containing hydrogen peroxide (maximum concentration 6%), or chemicals that release hydrogen peroxide (carbamide peroxide, zinc peroxide). Products come in different concentrations, and the higher the concentration the more likely the patient will experience sensitivity. European Union law forbids the use of products containing more than 6% hydrogen peroxide.

Patients can experience sensitivity when undertaking whitening, but this is transient and can be easily managed by the use of sensitive formula toothpastes or remineralising pastes/gels/mousse, such as GC Tooth Mousse® (which contains Recaldent™).

The gel is applied in the dental surgery or using custom-made trays at home. The process takes 2–3 weeks, but longer if the tooth shade is towards the blue/grey range. Whitening will not change the colour of crowns or restorations, and so if the patient is to undergo treatment to replace these, whitening should be undertaken first. It can, however, help with stains around the margins of restorations. The consumption of tea, coffee, red wine, turmeric, and tobacco should be avoided during the whitening treatment.

Patients should be advised that teeth whitening is not permanent. It can last anything from a few months to up to 3 years. Generally, the effect will not last long if the patient smokes, drinks red wine, tea, or coffee in significant amounts, which will all restain the teeth.

PLAQUE, CALCULUS, AND STAINING

REFERENCE

1. General Dental Council. (2018). *Tooth Whitening*. Available at: http://www.gdc-uk.org/patients/illegal-practice/legal-position [accessed 13 March 2019].

Chapter 3

Dental plaque-induced gingivitis

Learning outcomes

By the end of this chapter you should be able to:

1. Define dental plaque-induced gingivitis (and inflammation), and describe its primary and secondary causes.
2. Explain the difference between *signs* and *symptoms*, and list the signs and symptoms of dental plaque-induced gingivitis.
3. Explain how to treat this common condition.

DENTAL PLAQUE-INDUCED GINGIVITIS

Dental plaque-induced gingivitis (Figures 3.1, 3.2, and 3.3) describes the inflammation of the gums as defined in the *2017 Classification of Periodontal Diseases*. (It was formerly referred to as *chronic gingivitis* under the previous classification of periodontal diseases.)

Who does it affect?

Dental plaque-induced gingivitis is the condition that the oral health educator (OHE) will probably encounter most frequently in both children and adults.

In the UK Adult Dental Health Survey (2009), gingival bleeding on probing (a sign of active gingival disease) was found in 54% of dentate adults [1]. In the same survey, 59% of dentate adults aged 45–54, and 49% of dentate adults aged 65–74, showed gingival bleeding [1].

Since, initially, the condition rarely causes pain and affected gums can appear relatively normal, many sufferers are unaware that anything is wrong,

Basic Guide to Oral Health Education and Promotion, Third Edition.
Alison Chapman and Simon H. Felton.
© 2021 John Wiley & Sons Ltd. Published 2021 by John Wiley & Sons Ltd.
Companion website: www.wiley.com/go/felton/oralhealth

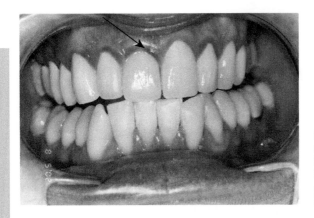

Figure 3.1 Localised marginal gingivitis. Source: Professor Nicola West, Bristol University. Reproduced with permission of Professor Nicola West.

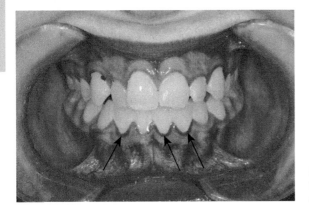

Figure 3.2 Generalised marginal gingivitis. Source: Alison Chapman.

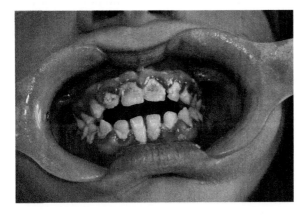

Figure 3.3 Gingivitis in a neglected mouth. Source: Alison Chapman.

and often will tell the educator that their gums have bled when brushing for years. OHEs will hear comments, such as: '*I thought it was normal for my gums to bleed*,' or, '*My gums always bleed when I have a new toothbrush*'.

The OHE should promote the message that, '*healthy gums do not bleed*', and in order to do this the educator needs to understand gingivitis and its causes, and have a basic knowledge of the body's inflammatory process.

Primary cause of dental plaque-induced gingivitis

The primary cause of dental plaque-induced gingivitis is simply poor oral hygiene; the bacterial by-products (i.e. enzymes and toxins) produced by mature plaque have the potential to directly damage the gingival tissue and also initiate inflammatory and immunological reactions in the tissues.

Secondary causes of dental plaque-induced gingivitis

Secondary factors increase the risk of the dental plaque, causing disease to the gingival tissues. They can be local (i.e. increasing plaque retention in a specific area), or systemic (whole body) conditions that alter the body's response to inflammation.

Local factors include:

- Malpositioned teeth.
- Overhanging fillings.
- Ill-fitting crowns, bridges, or dentures.
- Implants.
- Orthodontic appliances.
- Calculus.
- Lip apart posture (*mouth breathing*). The dryness of the attached gingivae in people whose lips are naturally parted when relaxed increases the likelihood of plaque retention.

Systemic factors include:

- Hormone changes during:
  - Pregnancy (pregnancy gingivitis) – swollen papilla, may progress to a pregnancy epulis (see Chapter 20).
  - Puberty (puberty gingivitis) – caused by testosterone, for example.
  - Menopause.
- Drug-induced:
  - Anticonvulsants (for epilepsy) – e.g. phenytoin and phenobarbital.

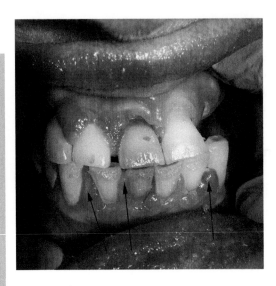

Figure 3.4 Drug-induced gingival growth (immunosuppressants for rheumatoid arthritis). Source: Alison Chapman.

- Immunosuppressants (anti-rejection medication for transplant patients) – e.g. cyclosporine (Figure 3.4).
- Certain calcium channel blockers (for high blood pressure) – e.g. nifedipine, verapamil, and diltiazem.
- Deep overbite causing direct gingival trauma.

Inflammation

The OHE needs a basic knowledge of the body's inflammatory process in order to explain gingivitis to patients who need to deal with the condition. When a word ends in '*itis*', it usually describes an inflammatory condition of a body tissue. For example, tonsill*itis* is inflammation of the tonsils.

Inflammation is the response of a tissue to injury, and is the first process by which the body defends itself against attack from:

- Physical sources (e.g. a blow to the mouth or a scratch from a toothbrush bristle).
- Chemical sources (e.g. an aspirin burn or a reaction to chemicals used in dentistry).
- Microorganisms (e.g. invasion by bacteria, viruses, or fungi).

Stages of inflammation (also signs of gingivitis)

The four stages of inflammation are also signs of gingivitis that the dental professional may notice:

1. Redness (*rubor*) – due to increased blood flow.
2. Swelling (*tumor*) – tissue fluid accumulates.
3. Heat (*calor*) – tissue temperature increases.
4. Pain (*dolor*) – rare in gingivitis, but some patients may complain of sore gums.

The words in brackets are Latin and they may help in remembering these stages by association (ruby from *rubor*; tumour from *tumor*; calories from *calor*, and doleful from *dolor*).

Other signs and symptoms of gingivitis

Signs are what the dental professional notices on examination, *symptoms* are what the patient may complain of. Both signs and symptoms of gingivitis are reversible and will disappear if inflammation is resolved by improved oral hygiene.

Signs
The dental professional may notice:

- Loss of stippling – the *orange peel* appearance seen in healthy attached gingivae, caused by bundles of collagen fibres beneath the epithelium. The inflammatory process damages these bundles and stippling disappears.
- Rounding of the gingival margin.
- False pocketing – caused by swelling of the marginal gingivae. There is no breach of the junctional epithelium, so the periodontal ligament remains intact.
- Loss of contour – gingivae lose their pointed shape due to swelling.
- Loss of consistency – gingivae lose their firmness and become soft and spongy.

Symptoms
The patient may complain of:

- Red, swollen gums.
- Bleeding on brushing – this is often the first thing that patients notice. They may also mention that their gums bleed when eating crisp foods, such as apples, or they may find blood on their pillow in the morning.
- Halitosis (*fetor oris*) – 'My breath smells'. May be caused by bleeding, but more likely to be noticed in periodontitis when debris becomes trapped in pockets (see Chapter 4).
- Itching or pain (rarely) – usually from trauma of vigorous brushing with a stiff brush, or when another factor is present, such as hormonal changes during pregnancy.

Remember! *Signs* are what the professional notices, *symptoms* are what the patient complains of.

Treatment of gingivitis

Treatment should include:

- Oral hygiene instruction, encouragement, and motivation.
- Removal/good care of potential plaque-retentive sites.
- Fluoride – antibacterial effect, and can be applied via toothpaste or mouthwash.
- Chemical (chlorhexidine mouthwash).
- Regular monitoring, including scaling, polishing, and reinforcement of oral health instruction.

REFERENCE

1. The Health and Social Care Information Centre (2011) *Disease and Related Disorders – A Report from the Adult Dental Health Survey 2009*. The Health and Social Care Information Centre, Leeds.

Chapter 4

Periodontal disease

Learning outcomes

By the end of this chapter you should be able to:

1. Define *periodontitis* and list the primary and secondary factors in its development.
2. List the signs, symptoms, and features of the condition, and explain its management.
3. Define *necrotising ulcerative gingivitis* (NUG), its causes and treatment.
4. Define *peri-implant mucositis* and *peri-implantitis,* and their causes and treatment.

WHAT IS PERIODONTITIS?

Periodontitis (Figure 4.1) describes the inflammation and gradual destruction of the periodontium (the supporting structure of the tooth).

Slowly progressing periodontitis was previously called *chronic periodontitis,* and rapidly progressing disease was called *aggressive periodontitis.* However, it is now thought that they are variations of the same disease process.

Periodontitis may look like gingivitis, but can be distinguished by:

- Periodontal probing (depth of pocket is greater than 3 mm).
- X-rays, which show loss of bone support.
- Loose teeth (potentially).
- Damage is not reversible.

Remember! It is important that the oral health educator (OHE) can distinguish between gingivitis (the continual but superficial inflammation of the gingivae), and periodontitis (the destruction of the periodontium).

Basic Guide to Oral Health Education and Promotion, Third Edition.
Alison Chapman and Simon H. Felton.
© 2021 John Wiley & Sons Ltd. Published 2021 by John Wiley & Sons Ltd.
Companion website: www.wiley.com/go/felton/oralhealth

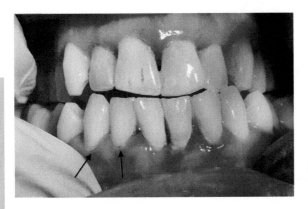

Figure 4.1 Adult periodontal disease. Source: Alison Chapman.

Who does it affect?

In the UK Adult Dental Health Survey (2009), only 17% of dentate adults showed no evidence of periodontal disease at the most stringent threshold [1].

Good periodontal health was more common among adults under 45 years old than in older age groups. For example, 20% of dentate adults aged between 25–34 years had very healthy periodontal tissues compared with 14% between 45– 54 years, and 10% above 55 years [1]. Twenty-one percent of dentate adults from managerial and professional occupation households had very healthy periodontal tissues compared with 16% of adults of intermediate occupations, and 12% of manual occupation households [1].

A growing body of research also suggests that there is an association between periodontitis and certain systemic (body) conditions, such as adverse pregnancy outcomes and type 2 diabetes [2].

Studies have also shown a link between periodontitis and coronary heart disease, and people with heart disease have an increased risk of periodontal disease. Acute coronary syndrome, high blood pressure (hypertension), and high cholesterol have also been associated with periodontal disease [3]. The more severe the periodontitis, the greater the risk of heart problems.

Primary causes of periodontitis

Periodontitis is often, but not always, a progression of gingivitis, and is primarily caused by the enzymes and toxins of mature plaque bacteria, which gradually break down the tissues of the periodontium in a susceptible host [4].

For most patients, gingivitis does not progress to periodontitis, but 10–15% of patients are susceptible to periodontitis [3]. The onset of periodontitis in these patients is thought to be due to a genetic abnormality, which causes a change in the behaviour of cytokines (substances which regulate the movement of immune system cells), and subsequent destruction of bone. This genetic basis explains why periodontitis frequently affects members of the same family.

Current thinking is that with periodontal disease, 20% of tissue damage is due to the direct effects of plaque by-products on tissues and 80% due to indirect effects, i.e. host destruction triggered by the body's own white blood cells [5].

Secondary risk factors in the development of periodontitis

Secondary factors are important in the development of periodontitis, and include:

- Smoking – the most important risk factor. Periodontal disease is more common in smokers than non-smokers [2]. Treatment response in smokers is also poorer than non-smokers. Smoking is thought to:
  - Reduce blood flow in the gingivae.
  - Reduce white blood cell mobility and function.
  - Impair healing.
  - Increase inflammatory substances (cytokines).
- Poor oral hygiene – failure to clean effectively, leading to plaque accumulation.
- Age – older people are more likely to have periodontitis, due to being exposed to plaque for a longer period than younger patients, and older people do not heal as easily.
- Plaque retention factors – poorly finished/worn fillings, dentures, crowns, bridges, partially erupted/impacted teeth, and supragingival/subgingival calculus (see Chapter 2).
- Crowding and malocclusion – one of the reasons for carrying out ortho-dontic treatment in childhood is to improve access to tooth surfaces and the ability to clean them, and prevent periodontal disease from occurring later. Bone loss associated with malocclusion is usually localised and not associated with poor oral hygiene.
- Carious cavities – plaque-retentive ledges.
- High frenulum insertion – usually found buccally on lower anteriors. The frenulum is a fold of mucous membrane, which limits the movement of the lower lip. If the insertion of the membrane is high on the gingivae, it can prevent effective oral hygiene and cause gingival recession.
- Systemic conditions (see Chapter 8) – for example, patients with diabetes, Down's syndrome, immunological disorders, and those who experience hormonal changes (e.g. during pregnancy and puberty).

Features of periodontitis

Features of periodontitis include:

- Often occurs in middle age.
- Usually progresses slowly.
- Can have unpredictable bursts of activity (active phases may need clinical intervention).

PERIODONTAL DISEASE

- Can result from the progression of gingivitis, but not always – many people have gingivitis for years but do not develop periodontitis.
- Patients can present with no obvious visual clinical signs (in some cases, the tissues can look quite healthy). Only pocket probing and radiographs will identify the loss of supporting structures.

Signs of periodontitis

Dental professionals in the UK have a duty of care to diagnose the disease in its early stages.

In the early stages of the disease, the dental professional will notice:

- A variable degree of gingivitis. Some patients still have gingivitis, others not.
- Bleeding on deep probing.
- The presence of subgingival calculus.
- Gingival recession.
- Bone loss – may be horizontal or vertical (and only apparent on X-rays).

In the advanced stage of the disease, the dental professional will notice:

- Periodontal abscess (see Chapter 8).
- Drifting and/or mobility of teeth due to loss of attachment (Figure 4.2). Fifty per cent of UK dentate adults over 16 years old have more than 4-mm attachment loss [1]. It is characterised by true pocketing (Figures 4.3 and 4.4), which may be either:
  - Suprabony (horizontal) – when the base of the pocket is above the crest of the alveolar bone.
  - Infrabony (vertical) – when the base of the pocket is below the crest of alveolar bone.

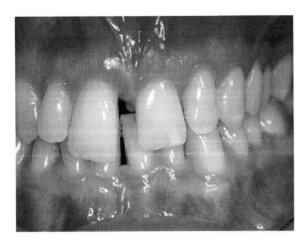

Figure 4.2 Drifting. Source: Professor Nicola West, Bristol University. Reproduced with permission of Professor Nicola West.

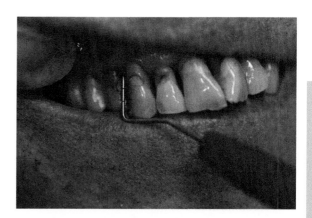

Figure 4.3 True pocketing, with probe inserted. Source: Alison Chapman.

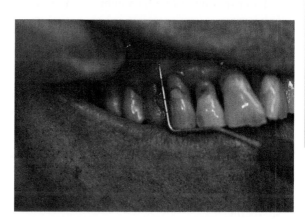

Figure 4.4 True pocketing. Source: Alison Chapman.

PERIODONTAL DISEASE

Symptoms of periodontitis

In the early stages of periodontitis, the patient may complain of:

* Recession – gums recede, and teeth may be hot and cold sensitive.
* Halitosis or a bad taste due to accumulation of bacteria in pockets and pus formation.

In the advanced stage of periodontitis, the patient may complain of:

* Drifting/mobility – loose/moving teeth.
* Pain (sometimes – from periodontal abscess).
* Pus oozing from pockets.

Treatment and management

Treatment and management of periodontitis includes the following:

* Encouragement and help to stop smoking (see Chapter 13).

PERIODONTAL DISEASE

- Regular maintenance and monitoring by:
  - Diagnosing and monitoring with pocket charting, bleeding indices (see Chapter 29), and removal of plaque retentive factors.
  - Effective regular plaque removal using manual or powered brush, and interdental brushes, plus (in severe cases) chlorhexidine mouthwash.
  - Toothpaste and mouthwashes containing fluoride are antibacterials and interfere with bacterial metabolism, reducing the number of bacteria present in the mouth.
  - Scaling, root surface debridement with ultrasonic scalers and hand scalers.
  - Air polishing – use of low abrasive agents, such as glycine or erythritol on the root surface to remove subgingival bacteria and reduce recolonisation.
  - Laser treatment in which light and a photosensitiser are used to destroy bacteria.
- Antibiotics – systemic or local.
- Chlorhexidine-impregnated chip placed in pocket.
- Surgery – re-contouring of gingivae and removal of pockets.

Remember! No periodontal treatment carried out by the dentist or hygienist will work if the patient does not maintain their oral hygiene.

Classification of Periodontal diseases
(Figure 4.5 a,b)

Periodontal diseases are classified by the British Society of Periodontology (BSP) by the:

- Extent – localised or generalised.
- Stage – ranging from stage I (early, mild) to stage IV (severe) using X-rays to measure the extent of interdental bone loss on the worst site (Figure 4.6).
- Grade – A, B, or C. Dividing the percentage of bone loss at the worst site due to periodontitis by the patient's age to determine the rate of progression of the disease.
- Current status of the disease – stable, in remission, or unstable.
- Risk factors – e.g. smoking, medically compromised.

NECROTISING ULCERATIVE GINGIVITIS

Necrotising ulcerative gingivitis (NUG) (Figure 4.7 a,b), also known as *acute necrotising ulcerative gingivitis* (ANUG), *trench mouth*, or *Vincent's angina*, is one of the most unpleasant acute illnesses to affect the oral cavity, and can make a patient feel extremely ill.

(a)

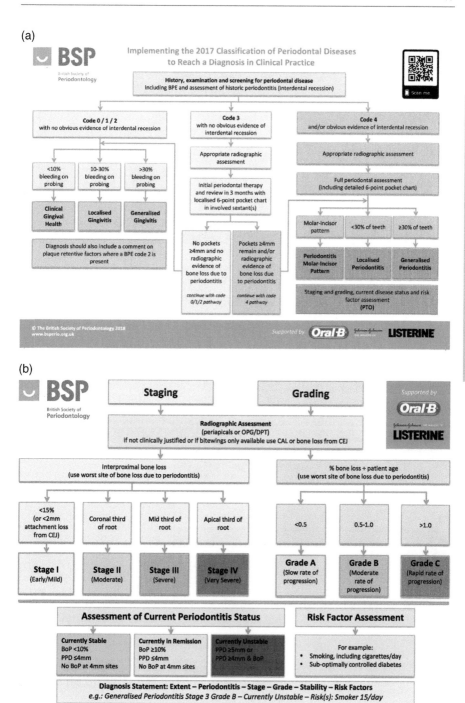

Figure 4.5 **(a,b)** Implementing the 2017 Classification of Periodontal Diseases to Reach a Diagnosis in Clinical Practice. Source: From [6]. Reproduced with permission of The British Society of Periodontology.

PERIODONTAL DISEASE

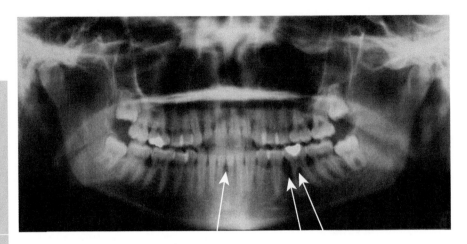

Figure 4.6 25-year-old woman; localised periodontitis, stage III (severe), grade-C, currently unstable, no risk factors. Source: Professor Nicola West, Bristol University. Reproduced with permission of Professor Nicola West.

(a)

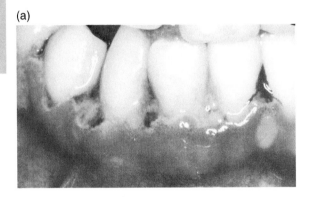

(b)

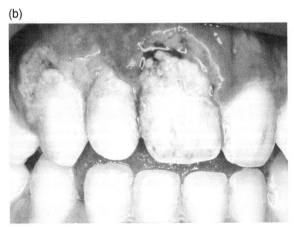

Figure 4.7 (a,b) Necrotising ulcerative gingivitis. Source: [7]. Reproduced with permission of Blackwell.

Aetiology of NUG

Causes of NUG are not fully understood – various microorganisms are involved, mainly anaerobic bacteria – the principle bacterium being *Treponema denticola*, which is capable of invading oral tissues [4].

NUG was common in the trenches during the First World War (hence the term trench mouth) and, although not contagious, tends to occur in communities where resistance is weak due to ill health or poor environmental conditions and nutrition.

Today, NUG is most commonly found in young adults between 18–25 years old, and often associated with students who have recently moved away from home and have started to look after themselves.

Predisposing factors include:

- Poor oral hygiene.
- Poor diet.
- Smoking.
- Immune system deficiency, such as HIV/AIDS.
- Stress/fatigue.

Clinical features of NUG

Clinical features of NUG include:

- Sudden onset and rapid development.
- Painfully inflamed gingivae and ragged, sloughing ulcers as bacteria invade the tissues.
- Acute inflammation and bleeding.
- Halitosis. Patients often complain of a metallic taste.
- Swollen glands, temperature, and general malaise.
- Destruction of tissues when no treatment is available – patients who have repeated attacks often exhibit permanent loss of interdental papillae.

Treatment of NUG

Treatment of NUG depends on its severity, but should be rapid to prevent the destruction of the interdental papillae, and includes:

- Stopping smoking and using recreational drugs (if applicable).
- Scaling – as soon as possible (on the first visit). An ultrasonic scaler makes the process quicker, gentler, and more tolerable for the patient.
- Hydrogen peroxide mouthwash – due to its mechanical cleaning properties and its ability to release oxygen into the area, killing the anaerobic bacteria.

- Chlorhexidine mouthwash – effective in reducing plaque formation as the patient may find it too painful to clean mechanically.
- Antibiotics (metronidazole, tetracycline) – if the patient shows signs of being generally ill with fever or severe lymph gland involvement.
- Emphasis on excellent oral hygiene.
- Reducing stress levels, regular rest.
- A healthy well-balanced diet (see Chapter 9).
- Regular dental appointments to treat and monitor the condition.

PERI-IMPLANT MUCOSITIS AND PERI-IMPLANTITIS

Peri-implant mucositis is a reversible inflammatory reaction causing redness and swelling localised to the soft tissue around implants.

Dental implants are used to replace missing teeth either on their own, as part of a bridge, or as an attachment for a denture. Modern implants have been used in dentistry since the 1960s (and are also used in other areas of the body for attaching prosthesis, such as in the ear).

The dental implant consists of a titanium screw placed in the bone of the maxilla or mandible, which is then left for up to six months to integrate with the bone before the final restoration is attached to it. They can be used to replace one tooth, as part of a bridge, or the foundation for a denture that either clips to the implant or is permanently placed. When designing the restoration, the ability to clean thoroughly around it should be considered as they can fail if excellent oral hygiene is not maintained.

The area around the junction between the implant and restoration is subject to gingival inflammation and bone loss just like a natural tooth with plaque and calculus accumulation. The depth of the gingival sulcus (gingival crevice) is deeper than that of a natural tooth and can be 3–4 mm.

Similar to gingivitis progressing to periodontitis, peri-implant mucositis can progress to peri-implantitis, which involves destruction of the bone (Figures 4.8, 4.9). The tissues around the implant should look similar to that of a natural tooth: pink, firm and stippled.

The patient should have regular dentist or hygienist appointments to assess, as early intervention in the event of a problem is important to prevent failure of the implant.

Oral hygiene aids for peri-implant mucositis and peri-implantitis

When advising patients on oral hygiene techniques, the depth of the sulcus must be taken into consideration.

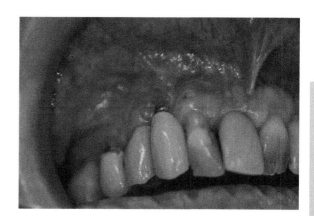

Figure 4.8 Peri-implantitis. Source: Alison Chapman.

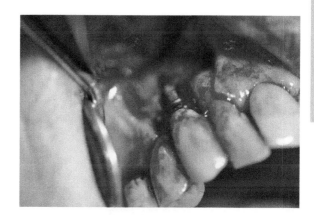

Figure 4.9 Peri-implantitis, surgically exposed. Source: Alison Chapman.

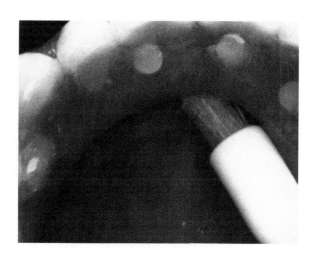

Figure 4.10 A single tufted or interspace brush, fixed lower. Source: Mary Mowbray. Reproduced with permission of Mary Mowbray.

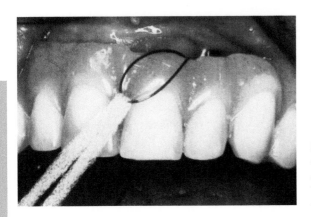

Figure 4.11 Floss threader on a fixed bridge. Source: Mary Mowbray. Reproduced with permission of Mary Mowbray.

(a)

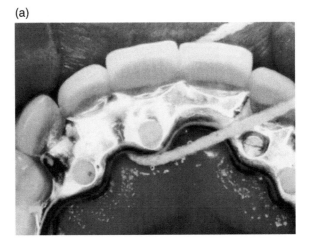

(b)

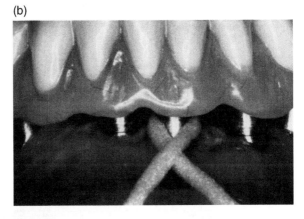

Figure 4.12 (a,b) Oral-B® SuperFloss™ with a fixed mix bridge (a) and fixed bridge (b). Source: Mary Mowbray. Reproduced with permission of Mary Mowbray.

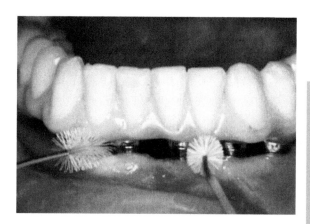

Figure 4.13 Interdental brush. Source: Mary Mowbray. Reproduced with permission of Mary Mowbray.

PERIODONTAL DISEASE

Oral hygiene aids include:

- An interspace brush (Figure 4.10) – this is used to clean subgingivally by flexing the tip and gently stroking it around the implant in the sulcus/gingival crevice.
- Dental floss, tape, floss threaders (Figure 4.11), Oral-B® SuperFloss™ (Figure 4.12 a,b), Tepe® implant floss – can be wrapped around the implant restoration and eased down into the sulcus. It should be wiped back and forth, or threaded under the bridge or denture, and moved along it to remove debris from underneath.
- Interdental brushes used in the same way as with a natural tooth (Figure 4.13).
- TePe® Implant Care™ brush – which is angulated to access the gingival sulcus lingually and palatally. It can be adjusted by warming in hot water, bending and then cooling in cold water.

REFERENCES

1. The Health and Social Care Information Centre (2011) *Oral Health and Function – A Report from the Adult Dental Health Survey 2009*. The Health and Social Care Information Centre, Leeds.
2. Greene, P.R., Jackson, M. (2012) The periodontium, tooth deposits and periodontal diseases. In: *Dental Hygiene and Therapy* (ed. S.L. Noble), 2nd edn, pp. 93–103. Wiley-Blackwell, Oxford.
3. British Dental Hygienists' Association (2006) *DH Contact*. British Dental Hygienists' Association, London.
4. Galgut, P. (2006) *Current Concepts in Periodontology*. Paper given at Gloucester Independent Dental Hygienists' Practical Periodontics Meeting. Cheltenham, Gloucestershire, 1 December 2006.

5. Van Dyke, T.E. & Serhan, C.N. (2003) Resolution of inflammation: a new paradigm for the pathogenesis of periodontal diseases. *Journal of Dental Research*, 82, 82–90.
6. The British Society of Periodontology (2017). *Implementing the 2017 Classification of Periodontal Diseases to Reach a Diagnosis in Clinical Practice*. Available at: www.bsperio.org.uk/publications/good_practitioners_guide_2016.pdf?v=3 [accessed 03 July 2019].
7. Claffey, N. (2003) Plaque induced gingival disease. In: *Clinical Periodontology and Implant Dentistry* (eds. J.T. Lindhe, T. Karring & N.P. Lang), 4th edn. pp. 198–208. Blackwell Munksgaard, Oxford.

PERIODONTAL DISEASE

Chapter 5

Caries

Learning outcomes

By the end of this chapter you should be able to:

1. Define *dental caries* and be aware of its history and incidence.
2. List sites where caries occurs.
3. Explain the development of caries.
4. Give simple advice to patients on preventing caries.
5. Conduct simple experiments to demonstrate how an acid attack occurs.
6. Describe studies linking caries to the consumption of fermentable carbohydrate.

WHAT IS CARIES?

Caries (a Latin word meaning *decay*) describes the progressive destruction of enamel, dentine, and cementum, initiated by microbial activity at a susceptible tooth surface.

The dental profession has been aware for many years that the frequency of sugar intake is far more significant in the development of caries than the amount consumed at any given time. Severe dental caries is likely to impair quality of life, including eating, speaking, sleeping, work/school, and can result in chronic systemic infection.

History of caries

The consumption of sugar in its various forms has long been associated with the development of caries.

In the UK, up until the seventeenth century, the diet consisted of unrefined whole foods, which wore occlusal surfaces flat. However, when fermentable

Basic Guide to Oral Health Education and Promotion, Third Edition.
Alison Chapman and Simon H. Felton.
© 2021 John Wiley & Sons Ltd. Published 2021 by John Wiley & Sons Ltd.
Companion website: www.wiley.com/go/felton/oralhealth

carbohydrates became an important constituent of the Western diet in the seventeenth century, people began to develop dental caries. Also, changes in flour-milling methods, which made flour more refined, meant that less chewing was required, and caries-prone fissures were not worn away. In the reign of Elizabeth I, sugar was imported and consumed by the wealthy. Dental caries became increasingly common following these changes in diet and as sugar became less expensive and more widely available to the general population.

Global incidence

In the present day, caries is one of the most widespread oral diseases found in industrialised countries, and the most common cause of tooth loss in both children and adults in the Western world (particularly in low socio-economic areas).

It is currently the most widespread non-communicable disease (NCD), and the most prevalent condition included in the 2015 Global Burden of Disease Study, ranking first for decay of permanent teeth (2.3 billion people), and 12th for deciduous teeth (560 million children) [3].

Nutritional changes in countries where there are inadequate oral health preventive measures (often unavailable in low- and medium-income countries), is associated with a marked recent increase in the burden of oral disease, including caries.

UK incidence (Dental Health Surveys)

According to the most recent Adult Dental Health Survey [1]:

- 24% of adults from managerial and professional occupation households had teeth with visible coronal caries (decay on crowns).
- 28% of adults from intermediate occupation households had visible coronal caries.
- 35% of adults from routine and manual occupation households had visible coronal caries.

Although our consumption of *visible* sugar is declining, it is increasingly found (hidden) in many processed foods, including confectionery, soft drinks, biscuits, and cakes (see Chapter 10).

In the Child Dental Health Survey 2013 (England, Wales and Northern Ireland), reductions were seen in the extent and severity of tooth decay using the dmft/DMFT index (see Chapter 29) in the permanent teeth of 12 and 15 year olds, when compared with the 2003 survey. There was also a reduction in 'obvious decay experience' in the permanent teeth of 12 and 15 year olds; in 2003, 43% and 56% saw decay, respectively, compared to 34% and 46% in 2013. Thirty five percent of 12 year olds and 28% of 15 year olds said they were, *'embarrassed to smile or laugh due to the condition of their teeth,'* and the burden of the disease remains considerable in those children [2].

CARIES

The 2013 survey also found that approximately 31% of 5 year olds and 46% of 8 year olds had obvious decay in their primary teeth. Untreated decay into dentine in primary teeth was found in 28% of 5 year olds and 39% of 8 year olds [2]. (It must be noted that figures from the 2003 survey cannot be compared with 2013 results due to the change in consent methodology for 5 and 8 year olds.)

Types of caries

There are three main types of caries:

1. Smooth surface caries (Figure 5.1).
2. Pit and fissure caries – common in newly erupted teeth (Figure 5.2).
3. Root caries – common in the elderly, when root surfaces are exposed (Figure 5.3).

CARIES

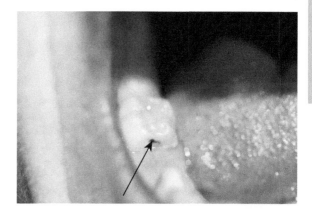

Figure 5.1 Smooth surface caries on lower molar. Source: Carole Hollins. Reproduced with permission of Carole Hollins.

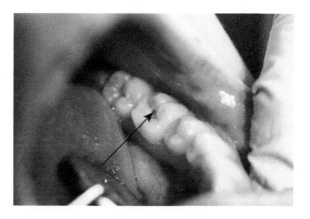

Figure 5.2 Pit and fissure caries on lower molar. Source: Carole Hollins. Reproduced with permission of Carole Hollins.

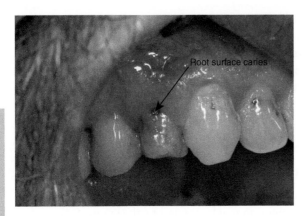

Figure 5.3 Root caries. Source: Dr Susan Hooper, Bristol University. Reproduced with permission of Susan Hooper.

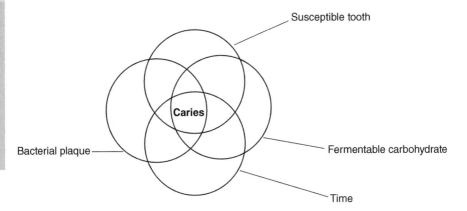

Figure 5.4 Causes of caries. Source: From Ruth McIntosh. Reproduced with permission of Ruth McIntosh.

Development of caries

For caries to develop, four factors are required (Figure 5.4):

1. Susceptible tooth.
2. Plaque.
3. Bacterial substrate (fermentable carbohydrate, which feeds plaque bacteria).
4. Time.

Remember! Susceptible tooth + bacterial plaque + substrate + time = caries.

Aetiology of caries

The normal (resting) pH of the mouth (and plaque) is around 6.7. This is neutral (i.e. neither acid nor alkaline).

When a susceptible tooth, often newly erupted (where the enamel has not yet matured), is exposed to frequent intakes of fermentable carbohydrates (starches that break down to sugars in the mouth), the bacteria present (most commonly *Streptococcus mutans* and *lactobacilli*) produce lactic acid and cause the pH of the mouth to drop. When the pH reaches 5.5 (known as *the critical pH*), an acid attack occurs [4].

High sugar consumption can result in an increased population of *S. mutans*, which can lead to a higher caries rate. If sugar consumption is reduced, the population of *S. mutans* will not always decline, leaving the patient with a higher susceptibility to caries.

Acid attack

During an acid attack, calcium hydroxyapatite in the enamel begins to dissolve as calcium and phosphate ions leave the tooth and pass into the saliva. This is the first stage in the development of caries, known as *demineralisation*.

Saliva contains bicarbonate ions, which have a buffering effect (neutralising acid), and if no more sugar is consumed, the calcium and phosphate ions return to the enamel and the pH returns to normal. It takes 30–60 minutes for this buffering to take effect and is known as *remineralisation*. Changes in the enamel surface during demineralisation and then remineralisation is known as the *ionic seesaw*.

When episodes of demineralisation exceed episodes of remineralisation dental caries can occur.

CARIES

The Stephan curve

The Stephan curve (Figure 5.5) is a graph used to show the development of an acid attack. It illustrates how quickly the pH falls and how long it takes to return to normal.

Remember! The role of bacterial plaque in the development of caries is that it:

- Maintains the concentration of acid at the tooth surface.
- Resists salivary buffering.
- Provides carbohydrate substrate (food for bacteria).

Stages of caries

The development of caries occurs in five stages:

1. Small pit – an initial break in the enamel extends to the enamel/dentine junction. It can be detected by a probe.
2. Blue/white lesion – caries destroys dentine more rapidly than enamel because it is softer. The decay shows through the translucent enamel as a blue/white area (Figure 5.6).
3. Open cavity – the unsupported enamel collapses (Figure 5.7).

CARIES

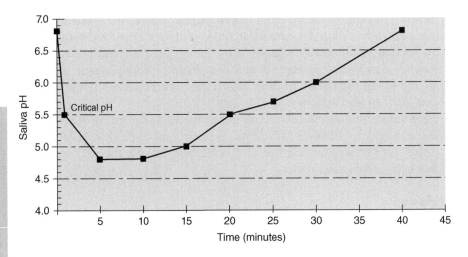

Figure 5.5 The Stephan curve. Source: From Ruth McIntosh. Reproduced with permission of Ruth McIntosh.

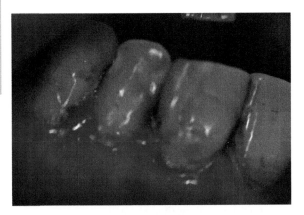

Figure 5.6 Blue/white lesion. Source: Alison Chapman.

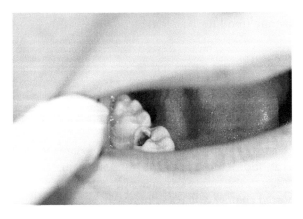

Figure 5.7 Open cavity. Source: [5]. Reproduced with permission of Wiley Blackwell.

4. Pulpitis – when the pulp cavity is reached, pulp becomes inflamed and pain occurs.
5. Apical abscess – infection spreads through the apical foramen into the periodontal ligament. Pulp is now dead, and the tooth is non-vital. Infection develops at the apex of the tooth, which can result in swelling. (This differs from a periodontal abscess, which forms on the side of the tooth.)

Common sites where caries occurs

The most common sites where caries occurs are:

- Occlusal surfaces, and buccal pits and fissures of newly erupted molars and premolars.
- Contact areas between adjacent teeth.
- Exposed root surfaces.
- Cervical surfaces at the tooth/gingival junction.

Prevention of caries (Figure 5.8)

Patients should be advised to:

- Cut down on refined sugars (particularly in sticky and liquid form).
- Restrict sugar to mealtimes.
- Brush twice daily with a fluoride toothpaste and spit, but not rinse.
- Clean daily interdentally, before brushing.

(For more detailed advice on sugars and consumption in preventing caries, see Chapter 10, and for details on the roles of fluoride and fissure sealants in preventing caries, see Chapters 11 and 12.)

CARIES

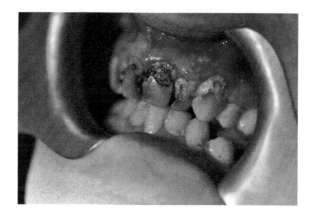

Figure 5.8 Gross caries in a neglected mouth. Source: Alison Chapman.

Simple experiments to demonstrate an acid attack

The following experiments are particularly effective for simulating an acid attack, which school children in particular may enjoy trying.

'Coins-in-acid' experiment

Fill seven plastic cups with: fizzy cola; orange juice; an isotonic sports drink; high-caffeine energy drink; orange squash; milk, and water. Take seven 1 or 2 pence tarnished copper coins and fix them to the cups with clothes pegs, so that half of the coin is immersed in the liquid and the other half remains dry. Leave the coins for an hour and observe the surprising results (as you may have expected cola to be the real *villain*). The neat orange juice and isotonic drinks will have lowered the pH more than the cola drink.

'Egg-in-fluoride' experiment

Fill an eggcup or one section of an egg box with fluoride toothpaste and plant an egg in it overnight (half the egg should be immersed in the toothpaste). The next day, remove the egg, mark the end which has been free of toothpaste with an indelible pen, and wash the toothpaste off. Immerse the egg in an acidic solution, such as white vinegar. Observe what happens.

You should have noticed that bubbles appear on the half of the egg not immersed in the toothpaste, indicating that the shell began dissolving in the acid and the fluoride in toothpaste has protected the shell from acid.

Epidemiology and caries

Epidemiology is the study of the incidence and severity of disease within population groups (see Chapter 29).

A number of studies have contributed to the existing knowledge of the causes and development of dental caries, including a recent Finnish study on xylitol (see Chapter 10), and two of the most important historic studies, the Vipeholm and Hopewood House studies.

The Vipeholm study

One of the most famous of all clinical dental studies began in 1939 when the Swedish Government requested an investigation to determine what measures should be taken to reduce caries in their country. This led to a study of the relationship between diet and caries, which took place at the Vipeholm Hospital near Lund in southern Sweden – an institution for people then described as, *'mentally diseased individuals'*.

The hospital, with its large number of permanent residents, provided an opportunity for a longitudinal study under well-controlled conditions.

A comparable study on human subjects will probably never be repeated, as it would now be regarded as unethical to alter diets experimentally in order to cause caries.

The patients were divided into seven groups: one control and six experimental. Four meals were eaten daily over one year, and all patients received a diet relatively low in sugar between meals. During this time, the number of new carious lesions was assessed and found to be very low [6].

After the first year, all but the control group were fed additions of large sucrose supplements in sticky or non-sticky forms, either with or between meals, and the results noted. The control group, which continued with the basic diet, showed little increase in caries throughout the study. In the experimental groups, the diet was supplemented by: sucrose in drinks; bread; chocolate; caramels; eight toffees, or 24 toffees a day. There was found to be a marked increase in caries in all experimental groups, except when the sucrose drink was taken at mealtimes [6].

The risk of sugar increasing caries activity was greatest if it was taken in sticky form between meals. In the 24 *toffees group*, when toffees were eaten between meals, the increase in caries was so great that the supplement was withdrawn [6].

UK dental professionals still base much of their dietary advice upon the results of this study, which ended in 1945, stressing that the frequency of sugar intake should be reduced and confined to mealtimes where possible. They advise against sticky foods and maintain that the rate of development of new disease will fall if their advice is followed.

Conclusions of Vipeholm study
At the end of the study, it was found that [6]:

1. Sugar consumption increased caries activity.
2. The risk of caries was greater if sugar was in sticky form.
3. Risk was greatest if sugar was in sticky form and taken between meals.
4. Increase in caries under uniform conditions showed great individual variation (therefore, other factors are involved).
5. Caries incidence reduces on withdrawal of sticky foods from diet.

Hopewood House study
In 1942, an eccentric and wealthy Australian businessman transformed Hopewood House, a country mansion in Bowral, New South Wales, into a home for children of low socio-economic backgrounds. Since this entrepreneur attributed his own improvement in health to dietary habits, he stipulated that the children should be raised on a natural diet excluding refined carbohydrates.

This environment provided the ideal opportunity for a dental study to take place, and at the time of the study 81 children were living in Hopewood House.

They were well fed, well clothed and had daily supervised exercise. All the children previously had poor oral hygiene, as this aspect of their health was not attended to and there was no fluoride in the drinking water.

Conclusions of Hopewood House study

At the end of the study, it was found that [7]:

1. Sixty-three of the 81 children were caries-free.
2. No child had more than six lesions.
3. All lesions were small.
4. Rates of initiation of new lesions and progress of established lesions were very much below the rates of the general population.
5. The difference between these children and the general population was the absence of refined carbohydrate.
6. Upon leaving Hopewood, their caries rate rose to the same level as the general population.

Other evidence-based studies

Other studies that show the relationship between sugar consumption and caries include:

- Toverund – a Norwegian World War II study when sugar was in short supply. There was a drop in the caries rate.
- Tristan da Cunha – a remote, untouched island in the South Atlantic until the 1940s when a fish-canning factory was built. Jams, cakes, and sweets were imported following an increase in the islanders' wealth. Prior to this event, islanders ate only what they grew or caught themselves. A survey in 1962 noticed that caries incidence had tripled since 1937 due to increased sugar consumption.
- Gnotobiotic (germ-free) rats – a laboratory study in which rats were fed varying amounts of sugar and their caries rate noted. It was found that germ-free rats fed on high levels of sugar did not develop caries – proving the need for bacteria to be present for caries to develop [6].
- Sweetened medicines – various studies of children on long-term medication have shown that sugared medicines cause higher caries rates [7].

CARIES

REFERENCES

1. The Health and Social Care Information Centre (2011) *Oral Health and Function – A Report from the Adult Dental Health Survey 2009*. The Health and Social Care Information Centre, Leeds.
2. NHS Digital (2015) *Child Dental Health Survey 2013, England, Wales and Northern Ireland*. Available at: https://digital.nhs.uk/data-and-information/publications/

statistical/children-s-dental-health-survey/child-dental-health-survey-2013-england-wales-and-northern-ireland [accessed 18 March 2019].
3. World Health Organization (2017) *Sugars and dental caries – WHO Technical Information Note.* Available at: www.who.int/oral_health/publications/sugars-dental-caries-keyfacts/en/ [accessed 20 March 2019].
4. Levine, R.S. & Stillman, C.R. (2009) *The Scientific Basis of Oral Health Education.* 6th edn. British Dental Journal, London.
5. Hollins, C. (2008) *Basic Guide to Dental Procedures.* Wiley-Blackwell, Oxford.
6. Fejerskov, O. & Kidd, E. (2004) *Dental Caries: The Disease and Its Clinical Management.* Blackwell Munksgaard, Oxford.
7. Health Education Authority. (1999) *Sugars in the Diet.* Health Education Authority, London.

Chapter 6

Tooth surface loss and sensitivity

Learning outcomes

By the end of this chapter you should be able to:

1. Distinguish between the three main types of tooth surface loss (TSL).
2. Describe the causes, features, and management of TSL.
3. Explain the causes of, and describe the treatment for, *sensitive dentine*.

WHAT IS TOOTH SURFACE LOSS?

Tooth surface loss (TSL) describes the loss of dental hard tissue when bacterial action (e.g. in caries) is not a factor.

There are three main types of TSL:

- Erosion.
- Attrition.
- Abrasion.

Incidence of TSL

The 2013 Children's Dental Health Survey found that 33% of 5 year olds, *'had evidence of TSL on one or more of the buccal surfaces of the primary upper incisors'*, and, *'TSL of the lingual surfaces was more common, with 57% of 5 year olds being affected'* [1].

The Survey also found, *'25% of 12 year olds had TSL on molars and buccal surfaces of incisors,'* and TSL on permanent incisors was more common on lingual surfaces than buccal surfaces.

Basic Guide to Oral Health Education and Promotion, Third Edition.
Alison Chapman and Simon H. Felton.
© 2021 John Wiley & Sons Ltd. Published 2021 by John Wiley & Sons Ltd.
Companion website: www.wiley.com/go/felton/oralhealth

The 2009 Adult Dental Health Survey showed that the prevalence of TSL in England had increased since the previous survey 10 years earlier, particularly in moderate TSL where values had risen from 11% in 1998 to 15% in 2009 [2].

Erosion

Erosion (Figure 6.1 a,b) is usually seen on occlusal, palatal, and lingual surfaces of anterior teeth, and sometimes on cervical margins. Dental professionals are seeing much more erosion in recent years and there are a number of reasons for this, mainly associated with modern lifestyles.

TOOTH SURFACE LOSS AND SENSITIVITY

(a)

(b)

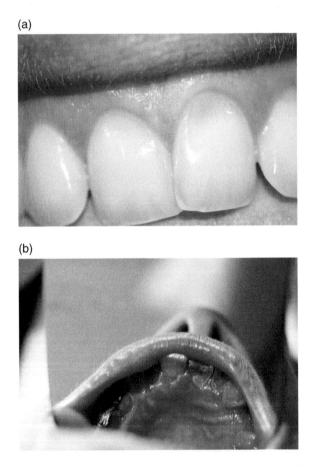

Figure 6.1 (a) Erosion on labial surface of upper incisors. Source: Carole Hollins. Reproduced with permission of Carole Hollins. (b) Erosion on palatal surface of upper incisors. Source: [3]. Reproduced with permission of Wiley-Blackwell.

Aetiology

Erosion is almost always associated with high acidity, which can be caused by factors, including:

- Diet. Often through frequent sipping of carbonated drinks or regular consumption of:
  - Citrus fruits/drinks, including fruit teas. The recommended '5-a-day' fruit and vegetable intake in the UK, whilst commendable for general health reasons, can encourage people to eat acid-rich fruits between meals and contribute to erosion.
  - Alcohol.
  - Some sports drinks.
  - Pickles.
- Regurgitation of stomach acids. Commonly seen in alcoholics, anorexics and bulimics, pregnant patients, or in people with chronic gastric disorders. Hydrochloric acid is responsible in these cases.

Features

Features of erosion include:

- Affected surfaces have a smooth, polished appearance.
- Where an amalgam filling is present, the tooth surface can reduce around it leaving a raised filling. Anatomical shape is lost, or shallow depressions may appear.

Patients commonly affected by erosion

Patients commonly affected by erosion include:

- Teenagers who sip carbonated drinks.
- Sports players who frequently drink *isotonic* drinks.
- Those with hiatus hernia/similar disorders, which cause acid regurgitation.
- Those with anorexia, bulimia, and pregnant women who vomit regularly.
- People who regularly eat citrus fruits (e.g. grapefruit for breakfast, followed by vigorous and damaging brushing), or drink high volumes of citrus juices.
- Chronic alcoholics, where regurgitation may occur.
- Elderly or medically-compromised patients whose saliva is greatly reduced.
- Preschool children with poor diets and oral hygiene.

Management/treatment

Management of erosion involves:

- Modifying diet (if diet-related). Particularly restricting acidic foods and drinks (and to regular mealtimes).
- Gentle toothbrushing – allow 2 hours after consuming acidic foods or drinks. Do not brush immediately after vomiting.

- Fluoride application – to increase tooth resistance to acid (e.g. Colgate Duraphat® 2800 or 5000, prescribed).
- Application of topical creams (e.g. GC Tooth Mousse®).
- Desensitising agents and toothpastes.
- Managing/treating underlying disorders.
- Reconstructing affected teeth.

Tooth surface loss through erosion can be monitored by the Basic Erosive Wear Examination (BEWE) Index (Table 6.1). If the affected teeth show signs of staining, then erosion is no longer happening as stains would be washed away by the acids.

The examination is repeated for all teeth in a sextant, but only the surface with the highest score is recorded for each sextant.

Attrition

Attrition (Figure 6.2) describes the wear seen on the crown of the tooth caused by friction from tooth-to-tooth contact, and is often seen on occlusal or incisal surfaces. It is common in older patients whose teeth have seen more wear and in the deciduous dentition where teeth are relatively soft. Some children grind their deciduous teeth so heavily that a tooth can be worn to almost nothing.

Table 6.1 Basic Erosive Wear Examination (BEWE) – criteria for grading erosive wear

Score	Wear
0	No tooth wear.
1	Initial loss of surface texture.
2*	Distinct defect (hard tissue loss <50% of surface area).
3*	Hard tissue loss (≥50% of the surface area).

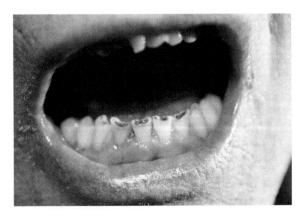

Figure 6.2 Attrition. Source: [4]. Reproduced with permission of Wiley-Blackwell.

Aetiology
Causes of attrition include:

- Bruxism (grinding or clenching).
- Diet (abrasive whole foods).
- Occupational (rare) – where abrasive dust is mixed with saliva (e.g. mining).

Features
Features of attrition include:

- Matching wear on occluding surfaces.
- Shiny facets on amalgam contacts.
- Enamel and dentine wear at the same rate.
- Possible fracture of cusps or restorations.

Patients commonly affected by attrition
Patients commonly affected by attrition include:

- Persistent grinders (often during sleep – a symptom of stress).
- Patients who eat a diet high in abrasive whole foods.
- Certain occupations (e.g. miners) with high exposure to abrasive dust.

Management/treatment
The management of attrition is the same as erosion, plus the use of a bite-raising splint at night.

Abrasion

Abrasion (Figure 6.3) describes the progressive loss of hard tissue due to mechanical factors other than tooth-to-tooth contact, i.e. exogenous (*outside*) factors of the oral cavity.

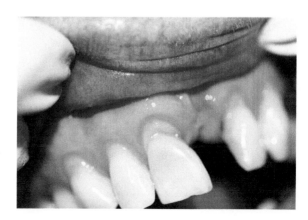

Figure 6.3 Abrasion cavities in upper incisors. Source: Carole Hollins. Reproduced with permission of Carole Hollins.

Aetiology

Causes of abrasion include:

- Destructive toothbrushing techniques.
- Pipe smoking – holding the pipe between the teeth.
- Oral and facial piercing – the ring or stud in the piercing can cause wear to the hard and soft tissues of the oral cavity (Figure 6.4).
- Occupational (e.g. pens, hairgrips, and tacks frequently held in mouth).
- Saliva combined with abrasive dust (rare, as with attrition).

Features

Features of abrasion include:

- Worn, shiny, often yellowy/brown-stained areas at cervical margins when aggressive toothbrushing is the cause, or on *biting surfaces* of anterior teeth in pipe smokers.

Patients commonly affected by abrasion

Patients commonly affected by abrasion include:

- Aggressive toothbrushers.
- People who use very hard toothbrushes.
- People with oral/facial piercing.
- Pipe smokers.
- People who persistently hold foreign objects in the teeth (e.g. hairdressers holding hairpins in their mouths).

Increasingly, professionals are seeing younger adults with abrasion. This obviously cannot be due to the wear of many years, and it is recognised that the Western diet is less abrasive in modern times. In younger people, it is more likely to be due to grinding and overzealous brushing with large amounts of toothpaste [2]. Some people are obsessed with having white teeth and brush overenthusiastically

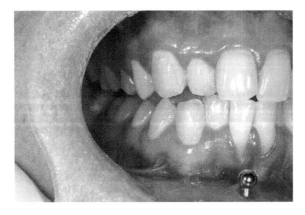

Figure 6.4 Oral piercing causing abrasion to the tooth and gingival recession. Source: Dr Nick Claydon. Reproduced with permission of Dr Nick Claydon.

several times a day. This can lead to TSL – the teeth appearing darker – and lead the patient to perpetuate the cycle by brushing even harder.

Management/treatment

- As with erosion, plus removal of piercing/replace with plastic version.

SENSITIVITY (DENTINE HYPERSENSITIVITY)

Sensitivity, also known as dentine hypersensitivity (DH or DHS), is an increasingly common chronic dental condition characterised by short, sharp pain arising from exposed dentine in response to external stimuli.

Dentine is a highly sensitive tooth tissue, and tooth sensitivity is often complained of by patients who think that they have developed a cavity or lost a filling. On examination, there is often no obvious reason for their pain, although gingival recession is sometimes apparent.

The amount of recession does not appear to be related to the incidence of sensitivity. Patients with large areas of exposed root are often symptom free, whereas patients with a minimal amount of exposed root sometimes suffer more.

Aetiology

Various theories have been put forward as to the causes of dentine hypersensitivity, but the most likely cause is exposure of dentine by TSL or gingival recession that, in some patients, changes the fluid flow rate in dentinal tubules, which stimulates tooth pulp.

Cold and sweet foods, and prodding from metallic objects, can cause this fluid to contract, but heat results in the expansion of fluid in tubules. Patients who complain of sensitivity to heat describe a pain that develops slowly and lasts longer than pain produced by other stimuli.

Common stimuli include:

- Cold air.
- Hot/cold foods and drinks (e.g. ice cream, tea/coffee).
- Sweet foods (e.g. boiled sweets and toffees).
- Touch by metal (e.g. fork).
- Chemical (bleaching).

Symptoms

Patients complain of episodes of short, sharp, severe episodes of pain sometimes referred to as an 'electric shock'. Sensitivity can result in great distress for patients to the extent that they avoid certain foods and dislike cleaning their teeth with anything but tepid water.

Some patients find that episodes of dentine hypersensitivity occur and then stop for no apparent reason. The condition often improves over time as secondary dentine is laid down.

Where does dentine hypersensitivity occur?

The most common sites where dentine hypersensitivity occurs are the buccal and labial surfaces of cervical margins. The teeth most commonly affected are permanent canines and premolars (possibly due to overenthusiastic brushing).

Patients commonly affected by dentine hypersensitivity

Patients commonly affected by dentine hypersensitivity include:

- Young adults (15–35 years old).
- Females, possibly because they clean their teeth more often and enthusiastically.
- Patients with highly acidic diets (fruit, yoghurt, etc.).
- Patients who vomit regularly (e.g. those with bulimia, pregnant women and hiatus hernia sufferers).
- Patients with acid reflux.
- Patients with severe occlusal trauma.
- Orthodontic patients (occasionally).

Treatment

Dentine hypersensitivity is treated by the application of any of the following products in the practice:

- Dentine bonding agents/occluding agents/bioactive glasses.
- Fluoride varnish.
- Restorations – glass ionomers/resin-reinforced glass ionomers/compomers/composites/onlays.
- Laser treatment.
- Endodontics (root canal treatment).

Treatment at home includes:

- Desensitising or sensitive formula toothpaste. Seems to be most effective (probably because of its cumulative effect, and desensitising agents such as strontium or arginine that block tubules).

TOOTH SURFACE LOSS AND SENSITIVITY

- Patients with many sensitive teeth may find relief from using:
  - A fluoride mouthwash (dose: 0.2% solution, 5–10 mL daily – for 12 years and above).
  - Topical cream (e.g. GC Tooth Mousse) containing calcium and phosphate, which helps remineralise the tooth surface (not suitable for patients with a milk protein allergy).
  - Toothpaste with a higher fluoride content (2800 ppm for patients 12 years and above, 5000 ppm for patients 16 years and above).

REFERENCES

1. NHS Digital (2015) *Child Dental Health Survey 2013, England, Wales and Northern Ireland.* Available at: https://digital.nhs.uk/data-and-information/publications/statistical/children-s-dental-health-survey/child-dental-health-survey-2013-england-wales-and-northern-ireland [accessed 18 March 2019].
2. The Health and Social Care Information Centre (2011) *Oral Health and Function – A Report from the Adult Dental Health Survey 2009.* The Health and Social Care Information Centre, Leeds.
3. Hollins, C. (2008) *Basic Guide to Dental Procedures.* Wiley-Blackwell, Oxford.
4. Hollins, C. (2008) *Levison's Textbook for Dental Nurses.* 10th edn. Wiley-Blackwell, Oxford.
5. Hollins, C. (2013) *Levison's Textbook for Dental Nurses.* 11th edn. Wiley-Blackwell, Oxford.

Chapter 7

Xerostomia

Learning outcomes

By the end of this chapter you should be able to:

1. Define *xerostomia*.
2. List the reasons for its occurrence.
3. Explain ways of managing this condition.

WHAT IS XEROSTOMIA?

Xerostomia is excessive dryness of the mouth.

Aetiology

Xerostomia is caused by insufficient oral secretions.

A reduction in the amount or flow of saliva, which may occur for various reasons, causes the balance of the mouth to be upset, and contributes to dental disease.

There are a number of reasons why saliva may be reduced or why its flow varies, including:

- Age – saliva production and flow diminish with age.
- Prescription drugs – certain drugs used for allergies, asthma, depression, diabetes, epilepsy, high blood pressure, inflammatory conditions, infertility, nausea, and Parkinson's disease. (See Chapter 8.)
- Anxiety – many people will have experienced a dry mouth associated with panic – perhaps before a dental appointment(!) or public speaking.

Basic Guide to Oral Health Education and Promotion, Third Edition.
Alison Chapman and Simon H. Felton.
© 2021 John Wiley & Sons Ltd. Published 2021 by John Wiley & Sons Ltd.
Companion website: www.wiley.com/go/felton/oralhealth

- Acute illness – diarrhoea and vomiting can cause dehydration, resulting in a reduction in saliva production. Infectious diseases like mumps (inflammation of the parotid gland) have the same effect.
- Mouth breathing – at night, or in people with malocclusion, or chronic sinus problems.
- Salivary calculi – calcified stones, which are stored in salivary ducts.
- Sjögren's syndrome (see Chapter 8) – associated with autoimmune conditions, such as rheumatoid arthritis, in which the lubrication of mucous membranes is drastically reduced. Patients often complain of dry eyes as well as a dry mouth.
- Radiotherapy (for cancer) – to the head and neck can cause a reduction in flow.
- Removal of a salivary gland.
- Menopausal women.

Permanently dry mouth

In some patients, their salivary flow never returns to normal and they suffer greatly from the effects of a permanently dry mouth (Figure 7.1), which are:

- Increased caries risk. In the elderly, root caries can be associated with xerostomia (which can cause plaque build-up), when gingival recession is present. The root surface does not have enamel protection and is prone to demineralisation (see Chapter 5).

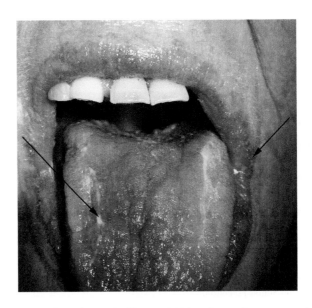

Figure 7.1 Xerostomia (note the cracked lips and thick, stringy saliva on tongue). Source: Alison Chapman.

XEROSTOMIA

- Gingivitis (sometimes leading to periodontitis). A reduction in salivary flow diminishes the self-cleansing ability of the mouth when the tongue has no lubrication to help remove stagnating food debris. This leads to more rapid formation of plaque and subsequent inflammation of the gingivae (see Chapter 3). The oral health educator (OHE) may have seen the bright red anterior gingivae of people with lip apart posture. This occurs because the anterior gingivae are permanently dry.
- Fungal and yeast infections. Organisms (e.g. *Candida*) proliferate in the dry mouth.
- Glossitis – sore tongue (see Chapter 8).
- Saliva is thicker, stickier and stringy.
- Altered or loss of taste.
- Tongue sticks to the roof of the mouth. This usually occurs at night when the salivary flow decreases further.
- Mouth burning sensation.
- Ulceration – particularly affects radiotherapy and chemotherapy patients, can be widespread, and exceedingly painful.
- Eating difficulties. Especially painful for radiotherapy patients with ulceration. Imagine trying to eat crisps, chocolate, or spicy foods with no saliva and a mouthful of ulcers.
- Speech difficulties.
- Denture sticking to the mouth.
- Altered oral sensation (mouthwashes and toothpastes may *burn*).

Salivary flow is also greatly reduced during sleep, which is why fermentable carbohydrates should not be consumed before bed (and after toothbrushing).

Management

Management of xerostomia depends on the cause of the condition.

For patients with chronic illness, who need to continue with their drug treatments, it may not be possible to remove the cause – so treatment in these cases is usually palliative. These patients should be advised to mention the problem to their doctor who may be able to alter their medication to help relieve symptoms.

All patients should be advised to maintain excellent oral hygiene to help with their symptoms. Plaque should be removed thoroughly by interdental cleaning and toothbrushing each day, and fluoride toothpaste and mouthwash used. High-fluoride toothpaste (2800 and 5000 ppm) is available by prescription.

The OHE can also advise specific toothpastes, which do not contain the foaming agent sodium lauryl sulphate that tends to dry the mouth, including some from the Sensodyne range, biotène®, bioXtra®, and Kingfisher.

Biotène and bioXtra sprays and moisturising gels (e.g. GC Dry Mouth Gel) are also options.

Gentle tongue cleansing is also advisable, as plaque will adhere more readily when it is not lubricated. Alcohol-free mouthwashes may also help.

Other measures that may help alleviate symptoms include:

- A diet high in fresh fruit and vegetables stimulates flow.
- Stop sugary snacks.
- Chewing sugar-free gum (containing xylitol) stimulates flow.
- Frequent sips of water or unsweetened drinks (non-alcoholic). Not fruit juices as these are high in acidity and can lead to erosion (see Chapter 6).
- Sucking small ice chips.
- Lubricating the mouth with non-virgin olive oil or sesame seed oil.
- Saliva substitutes available on prescription.
- Avoid smoking, acidic/spicy/salty foods, excessive caffeine/alcohol, and fizzy drinks.

Due to the number of management options available, the OHE should be able to discuss all of them with the patient to see which solutions suit them best, and advise the patient that they may need to use trial and error before finding the right solution(s) for them.

Management for radiotherapy/chemotherapy (and very ill) patients

Radiotherapy (receiving treatment in the head and neck area), chemotherapy patients and other very ill patients need extra special care to alleviate xerostomia, in addition to general management already mentioned.

Treatment is usually formulated by medical staff responsible for their care, and may include:

- Frequent, gentle cleaning procedures with specially designed soft swabs and (sometimes diluted) chlorhexidine gluconate mouthwash.
- Prescription drugs that stimulate salivary glands – e.g. pilocarpine (Salagen®).
- Use of artificial saliva substitutes available in sprays, toothpastes, gels and mouthwashes [1]. Be aware that certain products are artificially manufactured using pig's mucin and may not be acceptable to vegetarians and certain religious groups. These products are effective, but their beneficial effects are usually short-lived.
- Using a soft toothbrush/interdental brushes/sonic powered brush that do not cause trauma.

REFERENCE

1. Macmillan Cancer Support (2019) *Looking after your mouth during radiotherapy to the head and neck.* Available at: www.macmillan.org.uk/information-and-support/coping/side-effects-and-symptoms/mouth-problems/looking-after-your-mouth-during-radiotherapy.html#162969 [accessed 22nd March 2019].

Chapter 8

Other diseases and disorders affecting the oral cavity

Learning outcomes

By the end of this chapter you should be able to:

1. List disorders and diseases that affect the oral cavity.
2. Write brief notes on flash cards, summarising the main causes, features, and management of each (a good revision exercise for oral health education students).

INTRODUCTION

Many disorders and diseases affect the oral cavity. This chapter explores those, other than gingivitis, periodontitis, caries, tooth surface loss and xerostomia, which the oral health educator (OHE) may encounter, and includes their features, treatment and management. It includes certain systemic (whole body) conditions and diseases that can directly or indirectly affect the oral cavity.

PERIODONTAL ABSCESS

A periodontal abscess (Figure 8.1) is a localised collection of pus, also sometimes referred to as a lateral periodontal abscess, as it occurs on the side of the root or in the furcation (the division between two roots). It is usually, although not always, a development of advanced periodontitis.

Basic Guide to Oral Health Education and Promotion, Third Edition.
Alison Chapman and Simon H. Felton.
© 2021 John Wiley & Sons Ltd. Published 2021 by John Wiley & Sons Ltd.
Companion website: www.wiley.com/go/felton/oralhealth

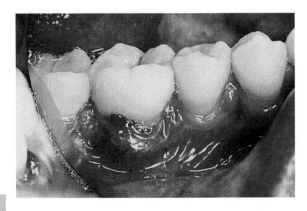

Figure 8.1 Periodontal abscess. Source: [1]. Reproduced with permission of Blackwell.

Aetiology (causes)

A periodontal abscess usually develops from a periodontal pocket, as organisms invade tissues and a foreign body or food debris blocks the outlet. It can still occur if oral hygiene improves before adequate scaling has taken place to remove the organisms (gingival tissue tightens as hygiene improves and stops pus oozing from the pocket).

Clinical features

Clinical features of a periodontal abscess, which may subside and recur, include:

- Swelling (sometimes localised, or the whole side of the face). This can also include localised swelling of lymph glands.
- Redness.
- Pain.
- Pus discharge (in later stages).
- Appears as a radiolucent (transparent) area on X-ray.

Treatment

Treatment depends on the severity of the periodontal abscess.
　　Short-term treatment includes:

- Hot saltwater mouth rinses.
- Antibiotics (often required) – topical (Dentomycin*), or systemic.
- Drainage – through deep scaling or incision.

　　Long-term treatment includes:

- Oral hygiene instruction – where the abscess occurs in the root furcation, the patient may be instructed to use an interdental brush through the furcation.
- Regular deep scaling (ultrasonic scaler) and irrigation (chlorhexidine).
- Extraction (last resort).

APHTHOUS ULCERS (MINOR AND MAJOR)

A mouth ulcer (Figure 8.2) is a painful open sore caused by a breach in the oral epithelium. Ulcers can occur for no apparent reason, are not contagious, and can affect the non-keratinised mucosa, lateral border of the tongue, floor of the mouth, buccal mucosa, and the lips.

Aetiology

The causes of mouth ulcers are not fully understood, but predisposing factors include:

- Trauma (e.g. from cheek biting, toothbrushing, hard foods).
- Orthodontic appliances.
- Inherited genetic susceptibility.
- Reaction to chemicals (e.g. sodium lauryl sulphate in toothpaste).
- Vitamin or mineral deficiency (B12, zinc, iron, folic acid).
- Hormonal (some women develop ulcers prior to menstruating).
- Gastrointestinal disease (e.g. Crohn's disease, ulcerative colitis, coeliac disease).
- Cow's milk allergy.
- Stress.

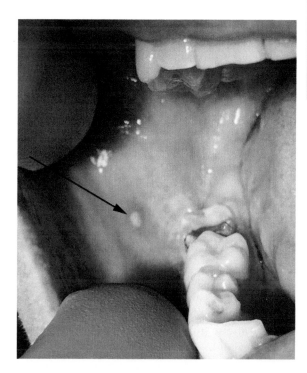

Figure 8.2 Mouth ulcer (apthous ulceration). Source: Alison Chapman.

OTHER DISEASES AND DISORDERS AFFECTING THE ORAL CAVITY

- Citrus fruits.
- Lack of sleep.
- Sudden weight loss.
- Immunodeficiency (e.g. HIV).

Clinical features

The following are clinical features of minor and major aphthous ulcers.

Minor aphthous ulcer

Clinical features of a minor aphthous ulcer include:

- Painful sore – a few millimetres in size. Red raised area around the border, with a white or grey centre.
- Circular or oval in shape.
- Can occur singularly or in clusters.
- Should heal after 7–14 days. If no improvement is seen after this time, the dentist should be consulted as this could be a sign of more serious disease, such as mouth cancer or gastrointestinal disease.

Major aphthous ulcer

Clinical features of a major aphthous ulcer include:

- 0.5–1 cm or more in size.
- Irregular shape.
- Can take up to 4–6 weeks to heal and can leave scarring.
- Often multiple, they can occur on keratinised and non-keratinised surfaces – lips, cheeks, and soft palate are common areas.

Treatment

There is no specific cure for major or minor aphthous ulcers, but patients can be advised on ways to alleviate the symptoms and pain as well as avoid known triggers:

- Use topical gels and sprays containing analgesics (painkillers) and local anaesthetic properties (e.g. Difflam™, Bonjela).
- Protection from secondary infection (consider chlorhexidine). Toothpaste free from sodium lauryl sulphate (e.g. Sensodyne® Pronamel™, biotene®, bioXtra®).
- Avoid spicy, acidic, or sharp foods.
- Control stress and get plenty of good quality sleep.
- A healthy, well-balanced diet (see Chapter 9).
- Silver nitrate (this burns the top layer of the ulcer, which reduces pain and aids healing).

- Mineral or vitamin B12 supplements.
- Orthodontic appliances (soft wax can be placed over the appliance where the ulcer forms).
- Herbal remedies and homeopathy – for example, aloe vera (in toothpaste), feverfew, and propolis ointment (see Chapter 19).

COLD SORES (HERPES LABIALIS)

Cold sores (Figure 8.3) are common, and most sufferers are infected in early childhood, often through close contact with a relative (kissing). When a small child is first infected, the disease can present as an acute and unpleasant illness (see primary herpetic gingivostomatitis).

Aetiology

Cold sores are caused by an infection with the herpes simplex virus at nerve endings. The virus can live throughout the life of an individual and reactivates. Contact with others (usually mouth) leads to the spread of the virus.

Clinical features

Clinical features (and contagious stages) of cold sores include:

1. Tingling in the area of eruption.
2. A small, raised blotch that forms blisters.
3. Blisters collapse – causing weeping.
4. Scab – blister dries and heals.

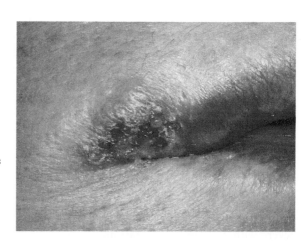

Figure 8.3 Cold sore (*herpes labialis*). Source: Professor M.A.O. Lewis, Cardiff University. Reproduced with permission of Professor M.A.O. Lewis.

OTHER DISEASES AND DISORDERS AFFECTING THE ORAL CAVITY

The cold sore is highly contagious until it has healed. Sufferers should avoid physical contact with other people while the cold sore is present (especially important with young children). They should also not attend dental appointments.

What reactivates the virus?

The virus is often reactivated by the following:

- Illness (e.g. cold, flu, AIDS).
- Emotional stress.
- Menstruation.
- Bright sunlight (which explains why some people develop cold sores while on holiday).
- Extreme cold weather.
- Fatigue and physical injury.

Treatment

Treatment of cold sores includes:

- Prescribed antiviral cream – should be applied at the initial tingling stage before clinical signs appear. Scratching or close contact with others (particularly young children) should be avoided.
- Severe cold sores can be treated using systemic antiviral drugs.
- Over-the-counter medicines, cold sore patches.
- Herbal remedies and homeopathy (see Chapter 19) – for example, propolis ointment.

PRIMARY (ACUTE) HERPETIC GINGIVOSTOMATITIS

Primary (Acute) herpetic gingivostomatitis (Figure 8.4), also known as primary gingival herpetic stomatitis, is how the herpes simplex virus can present in babies and small children, and it is occasionally seen in adults who have lowered immunity.

Aetiology

It is caused by infection with the herpes simplex virus.

Clinical features

The herpes simplex virus may be mild and produce few symptoms, or may be severe with widespread ulceration.

OTHER DISEASES AND DISORDERS AFFECTING THE ORAL CAVITY

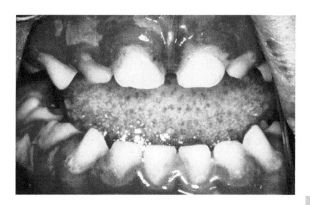

Figure 8.4 Acute herpetic gingivostomatitis. Source: [2]. Reproduced with permission of Blackwell.

Clinical features include:

- Small vesicles (blisters), which rupture and produce ulcers, appear in the mouth and/or throat.
- Sudden onset of feeling unwell and irritability.
- Dehydration (due to refusal to eat and drink).
- Dribbling – as too painful to swallow saliva.
- General malaise – fever, coated tongue, swollen tongue, and foul breath.

Treatment

It is treated as a flu-like illness, by:

- Rest.
- Frequent fluid, soft foods (infants may require hospital treatment to restore fluids if they refuse to drink).
- Mild analgesics.
- Chlorhexidine mouthwash (for adults).
- Gentle oral hygiene.
- Antiviral drugs (may be prescribed in severe cases).

TOOTH ANOMALIES

Hypodontia

Hypodontia is a congenital (i.e. *from birth*) disorder that describes a reduced number of teeth. It usually occurs in the permanent dentition and rarely in the deciduous dentition [3]. The teeth most commonly missing are lower third molars, upper lateral incisors, and lower second premolars. Hypodontia can be hereditary, but can also occur for no apparent reason.

Anodontia

Anodontia is a congenital disorder that describes the total absence of teeth. It is rare and usually associated with the hereditary genetic condition hypohidrotic ectodermal dysplasia (a genetic defect in which patients have very few or no teeth, and an absence of hair and sweat glands) [3].

Hyperdontia

Hyperdontia is a congenital disorder in which the person has more teeth than normal. The extra teeth are called *supernumerary teeth*. They can occur anywhere in the mouth, but are most commonly found anteriorly in the maxilla and in the premolar region of the mandible. They occur most frequently in the permanent dentition and in women, and can cause crowding, prevent teeth erupting, the displacement of teeth, and resorption if unerupted [3].

Supernumerary teeth are classified according to their morphology (shape), which are known as *supplemental* (including conical, tuberculate, molariform), and their location (mesiodens, paramolar, distomolar).

The most common type of supernumerary teeth are mesiodens (Figure 8.5), which occur between the upper central incisors. Paramolars are found in addition to molars.

Teeth size

Genetic factors can cause abnormalities in tooth size, causing them to be unusually large or small. The whole dentition is usually affected, but it occasionally affects just a few teeth. Peg-shaped upper lateral incisors can also herald a missing lateral on the opposite side.

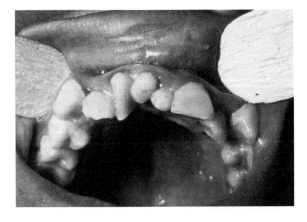

Figure 8.5 Two mesiodens in the midline between the upper central incisors. Source: [4]. Reproduced with permission of Wiley-Blackwell.

Tooth morphology anomalies

Variations in morphology of the tooth root or crown are quite common. They may present as [3]:

- Double tooth (Figure 8.6) – where two teeth have fused together during development.
- Enamel pearls – nodules on the buccal root surface.
- *Dens in dente* – literally a tooth within a tooth.
- Dilaceration (disturbance in tooth shape) – caused by trauma to the developing tooth resulting in the root and crown being bent.
- *Amelogenesis imperfecta* – an inherited disorder, in which the enamel is poorly mineralised and defective resulting in soft, brittle, and pitted enamel that can breakdown after eruption.
- *Dentinogenesis imperfecta* – a genetic defect of the dentine. There are two types:
  - Type 1 – occurs in association with *osteogenesis imperfecta*, in which there is a defective bone formation.
  - Type 2 – more common, and affects both the deciduous and permanent dentition. Although normal shape on eruption, the teeth have an amber-brown or purple-blue colour. The enamel breaks away from the underlying defective dentine.
- Enamel hypoplasia – a disturbance in the formation of enamel. It can affect a single tooth, be localised, affect several teeth or be generalised. It is caused by disturbances when the tooth is developing and usually occurs in the first 10 months of life or in the womb if the mother has a viral infection, such as measles or mumps, or due to excessive fluoride intake (see Chapter 11). It is common in children with low birth weight or systemic illness, and can result in yellowy/brown defects, white opacities, and pitted or irregular enamel.

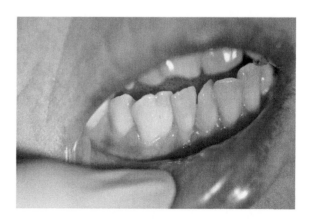

Figure 8.6 Double tooth.
Source: Alison Chapman.

OTHER DISEASES AND DISORDERS AFFECTING THE ORAL CAVITY

BURNING MOUTH SYNDROME

Burning mouth syndrome (BMS) is a painful and often persistent long-term condition, more common in women (particularly menopausal) and is thought to affect around 5% of the UK population, and can lead to a reduced quality of life [5]. There is no test for BMS and diagnosis involves ruling out other conditions with blood tests [6].

Aetiology

The exact cause of BMS is unknown, but some research suggests that it could be caused by underlying nerve damage to the tongue that changes the way the tongue transmits heat, cold, and taste to the brain, and results in neuropathic pain. Hormonal changes may also play a part [5-7].

Symptoms

There are no clinical features of BMS, but symptoms can include:

- Burning pain/hot sensation.
- Pain can be continuous or intermittent.
- Localized to lips or tongue, or more widespread in the mouth.
- Dry mouth.
- Unpleasant taste/changes to taste.
- Numbness.
- Depression/mood changes/fatigue (lack of sleep).

Treatment

There is no known cure for BMS (reviews on clinical trials have shown insufficient evidence), but patients may be prescribed the following treatments (and advised to avoid known triggers), which may help alleviate symptoms [6,7]:

- Antidepressants, antipsychotics, tranquillisers, saliva stimulants, and drugs for neuropathic pain.
- Dietary supplements.
- Directed energy waves.
- Cognitive behavioural therapy (CBT).
- Coping strategies, such as rest and relaxation techniques.
- Sipping cold water/sucking on ice cubes.
- Chewing sugar-free gum.
- Avoiding hot/spicy/acidic foods and alcohol [5].

OTHER DISEASES AND DISORDERS
AFFECTING THE ORAL CAVITY

GLOSSITIS

Glossitis (Figure 8.7) describes inflammation of the tongue.

Clinical features

In glossitis, the tongue becomes redder in colour and in some cases can swell (although rare, this may lead to hospitalisation and even a tracheotomy). In other cases, the dental papillae are lost, leaving a smooth surface. Sometimes, only a small area of the tongue loses its papillae, usually in the middle of the dorsum of the tongue.

Symptoms

Glossitis can be painless, but can also cause discomfort of the tongue and palate, leading to difficulty in chewing, swallowing, and speaking.

Aetiology

Causes of glossitis include:

- Bacterial or viral infections.
- Xerostomia (see Chapter 7).
- Irritation or injury – from burns, rough teeth, tobacco, alcohol, and spices.
- Allergic reaction – to toothpaste, mouthwash, breath fresheners, dyes in confectionery, plastic in dentures or retainers, and certain blood-pressure medications.
- Disorders – such as anaemia, vitamin B12 deficiency, oral lichen planus, and aphthous ulcers.
- Genetic (inherited).

OTHER DISEASES AND DISORDERS AFFECTING THE ORAL CAVITY

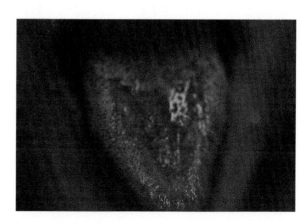

Figure 8.7 Glossitis. Source: Alison Chapman.

Treatment

Glossitis usually responds well to treatment, which includes:

- Removal of the irritant (if the cause).
- Antibiotics.
- Health check for deficiencies.

GEOGRAPHIC TONGUE

Geographic tongue is also known as *benign migratory glossitis* because its appearance is constantly changing. Although geographic tongue is benign (harmless), it may persist for months or longer, and often recurs.

Clinical features

Geographic tongue appears as irregularly shaped (*map-like*) smooth, red patches on the tongue where the papillae are missing (Figures 8.8, 8.9). A white border sometimes surrounds patches. Lesions are usually confined to the tongue, but they sometimes occur elsewhere in the mouth or on the lips.

Symptoms

In some cases, there are no symptoms, but burning or irritation of the tongue is common, particularly with hot or spicy foods. The discomfort may come and go over time and may worsen at certain times, for example, during pregnancy and menstruation.

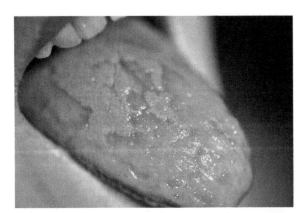

Figure 8.8 Geographic tongue. Source: Alison Chapman.

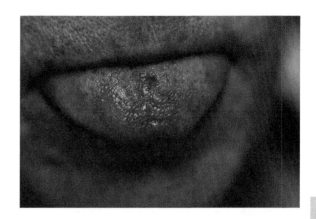

Figure 8.9 Geographic tongue (tip). Source: Alison Chapman.

Aetiology

The exact causes of geographic tongue are unknown, but it has been linked to:

- Patients with psoriasis.
- Coeliac disease, diabetes, anaemia, eczema, stress, and asthma. (Asthmatics should rinse their mouth after using their preventive medicine.)
- Trigger foods (in some patients) – e.g. cheese, fruits (raspberries, strawberries, and pineapple).
- Family history.
- The menstrual cycle (may be hormone related).
- Vitamin B12 deficiency.

Treatment

There is no known cure for geographic tongue, but pain may be relieved by:

- Using mouthwashes that contain a topical anaesthetic.
- Avoiding trigger foods.
- Blood tests for vitamin B12 deficiency and treatment accordingly.

BLACK HAIRY TONGUE

Black hairy tongue is a harmless condition affecting the papillae on the dorsum of the tongue (Figure 8.10). It is more common in men, usually affecting those over 40 years old. Although harmless, it can be alarming in appearance and patients may complain of burning, tickling, nausea, or halitosis.

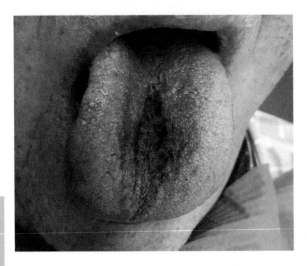

Figure 8.10 Black hairy tongue. Source: Alison Chapman.

Aetiology and clinical features

Defective shedding of the tongue's surface cells lead to long hair-like projections (up to 18 mm long) where bacteria and yeasts overgrow, producing discolouration (usually brown or black, but can be yellow or green), and food debris accumulates.

Other factors that may cause or aggravate the tongue, include:

- Smoking, chewing tobacco.
- Antibiotics.
- Alcohol.
- Cocaine.
- Mouthwash (chlorhexidine).
- Tea, coffee.
- Dehydration.
- Xerostomia (see Chapter 7).
- Radiotherapy.

Treatment

Treatment includes:

- Avoiding contributing factors.
- Good oral hygiene.
- Gentle brushing or tongue scraping.
- Mouthwash (containing hydrogen peroxide).
- Antibacterial mouthwash.

ORAL CANDIDOSIS

Candidosis is caused by the fungus *Candida albicans.* This fungus is commonly present in the oral cavity and usually causes no problems. However, as with many organisms, it can become active when resistance is low.

The most common manifestations of the fungus seen by the dental professional are oral thrush, stomatitis, and angular cheilitis.

It affects young babies, older people and the terminally ill in particular. Asthma sufferers are also prone to thrush, since the steroids in inhalers alter the oral flora. They should be advised to rinse their mouths out with water after using inhalers. Oral thrush can also occur after a course of antibiotics, which can affect the balance of the normal oral flora.

Oral thrush

Clinical features
Clinical features of oral thrush (Figure 8.11) include:

- Thick, white patches on the tongue, cheeks, lips, and palate.
- Red, raw, sore patches remain when the white coating is removed. This feature helps distinguish thrush from more serious conditions, such as oral carcinoma.

Treatment
Oral thrush is treated using antifungal drugs (e.g. Nystatin – systemic, pastilles, or oral suspension).

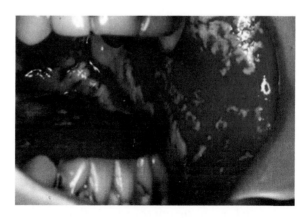

Figure 8.11 Oral thrush. Source: Professor M.A.O. Lewis, Cardiff University. Reproduced with permission of Professor M.A.O. Lewis.

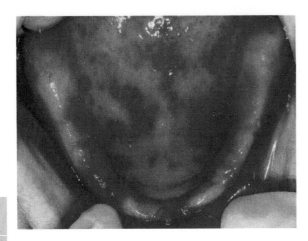

Figure 8.12 Denture stomatitis. Source: Alison Chapman.

Stomatitis

Stomatitis is a fungal inflammation of the mucous membrane lining of the mouth, and may involve the cheeks, gums, tongue, lips, and roof or floor of the mouth. It is usually associated with denture wearing, known as *denture stomatitis* (Figure 8.12) and/or antibiotic therapy. It may occur post-antibiotics.

Clinical features
Clinical features of stomatitis include:

- Red, shiny, sore patches, often on the palate or around the teeth where a denture fits.

Treatment
Treatment of stomatitis includes:

- Removal and brief sterilisation of dentures at night – if possible, or leave out for periods in the day.
- Avoidance of antibiotics (where practical).
- Antifungal drugs.
- Gentle brushing of affected areas.

Angular cheilitis

Angular cheilitis (Figure 8.13) is caused by a fungus or bacteria that results in cracks at the angles of the mouth. It is usually seen in older people or denture wearers where the mouth overcloses, thus keeping the areas continually moist, which encourages the proliferation of fungus or bacteria.

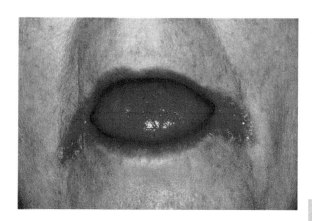

Figure 8.13 Angular cheilitis. Source: Professor M.A.O. Lewis, Cardiff University. Reproduced with permission of Professor M.A.O. Lewis.

Clinical features

Clinical features of angular cheilitis include:

- Small, reddened, sore cracks at angles of the mouth, which either do not heal, or continually recur.
- Dry lips.
- Burning sensation (on touch).

Treatment

Treatment of angular cheilitis includes:

- Replacement of ill-fitting dentures.
- Antifungal ointment (if cause is fungus) – which must be used for the prescribed length of time (i.e. for several weeks after infection has gone).
- A combination of mupirocin or fusidic acid, and 1% hydrocortisone cream (if cause is bacterial).
- Herbal remedies and homeopathy – for example, aloe vera (in cream), and propolis ointment (see Chapter 19).

WHITE PATCHES (LEUKOPLAKIA)

The majority of white patches seen in the mouth are benign, but certain conditions may be pre-malignant or malignant. It is, therefore, recommended that all white patches should be sent for biopsy.

There are a number of causes of leukoplakia (Figure 8.14) including:

- Smoker's keratosis.
- Trauma (such as cheek biting).
- Aspirin contact next to a tooth (some patients may do this if they have a toothache).

OTHER DISEASES AND DISORDERS AFFECTING THE ORAL CAVITY

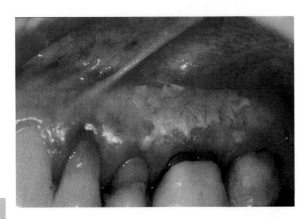

Figure 8.14 Leukoplakia (white patches). Source: Mary Mowbray. Reproduced with permission of Mary Mowbray.

ORAL CANCER (CARCINOMA)

Oral cancer (Figures 8.15, 8.16) is part of a group of cancers referred to as head and neck cancers (excludes the brain), of which mouth cancer accounts for approximately 85% of the group worldwide [8].

It can affect all of the soft tissues in the mouth and salivary glands, and the most commonly affected sites are the lateral borders (sides) of the tongue, floor of the mouth, and the retromolar region – to the sides of, and behind, the last molars (Figure 8.17).

There are around 12 000 cases of head and neck cancer diagnosed in the UK each year, it is the fourth most common cancer in males, and the highest incidence is in people between 70 and 74 years old. Most head and neck cancers occur in the larynx, its incidence has increased by 31% since the early 1990s, and it accounts for over 4000 deaths per year in the UK [9]. Most patients with lip cancer survive over 5 years. The percentage of people who develop cancer in the posterior parts of the mouth is relatively low.

Often, mouth cancer is only discovered when the cancer has metastasized to the lymph nodes of the neck, and is a major reason why patients should be screened regularly by a dentist (at least once a year) in order for early diagnosis and improving survival chances.

At each dental appointment, the dentist should undertake an extraoral and intraoral examination of the soft tissues, looking for any signs of cancer or other diseases. Various systems are available to test suspicious areas, including dyes and/or special lights to highlight areas that need further investigation (rather than being a diagnosis). The OHE is also in a prime position to notice lesions in a patient's mouth and should refer any suspicious findings to the dentist.

Aetiology

The causes of mouth cancer are complex, there is little evidence of genetic links, and environmental factors play an important part. Lifestyle factors, most

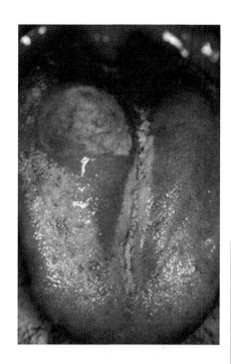

Figure 8.15 Oral cancer (tongue). Source: Professor M.A.O. Lewis, Cardiff University. Reproduced with permission of Professor M.A.O. Lewis.

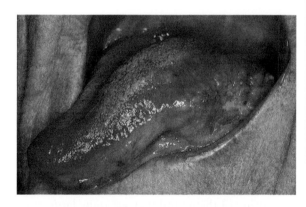

Figure 8.16 Oral cancer (base of the tongue). Source: Professor M.A.O. Lewis, Cardiff University. Reproduced with permission of Professor M.A.O. Lewis.

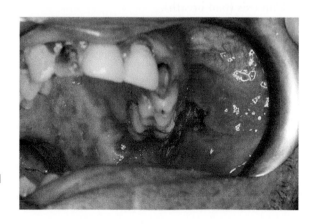

Figure 8.17 Oral cancer (retro molar triangle). Source: Professor M.A.O. Lewis, Cardiff University. Reproduced with permission of Professor M.A.O. Lewis.

notably tobacco and alcohol, have been linked particularly with cancer in the anterior part of the mouth, and research has shown that people who drink and smoke/chew tobacco have a 15 times greater risk of developing mouth cancer than others [8]. Cigarettes and alcohol contain nitrosamines and other chemicals that are known to cause cancer. Betel nut/paan chewing is also a high risk factor (see Chapter 13).

The disease (particularly in the posterior part of the mouth) has also been linked to the human papillomavirus (HPV) – a group of viruses that affect the skin. Most people will experience some type of HPV in their life, but it usually does not manifest into a problem and many are unaware of it. Schoolchildren (aged 12–13) are now offered vaccinations for HPV.

Research has also shown that excessive exposure to sunlight increases the incidence of lip cancers, although incidence of this type of cancer, which may present as dark patches or non-healing sores, has declined in recent years as we have become more aware of the importance of sun protection [8].

A diet low in fresh fruit and vegetables (and poor immune system) can also contribute to cancer development as these are valuable sources of antioxidants, which help prevent cell damage.

Clinical features

Clinical features of mouth cancer include:

- Red patches – can be speckled or have a velvety appearance.
- Non-healing ulcers – typically the ulcers have raised, rolled margins.
- White patches (leukoplakia).
- Lumps or nodules in the mouth, lip, or neck.
- Tissues firm or hard to touch.
- Loose teeth.
- Bleeding or numbness in the mouth.
- Lesions are usually painless in the early stages and many patients are unaware of them until they are quite large.
- Halitosis (bad breath).
- Significant weight loss in a short period of time.

Treatment

Treatment of mouth cancer includes:

- Surgery.
- Radiotherapy. Side effects of radiotherapy include xerostomia (see Chapter 7), leading to ulceration and increased caries rate.
- Chemotherapy (occasionally).
- Specialised palliative cleaning techniques – worked out by oncology care teams, plus the use of mouthwashes and other products. OHEs should be

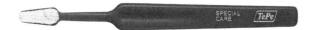

Figure 8.18 TePe® Special Care toothbrush. Source: TePe Oral Hygiene Products Ltd. Reproduced with permission of TePe Oral Hygiene Products Ltd.

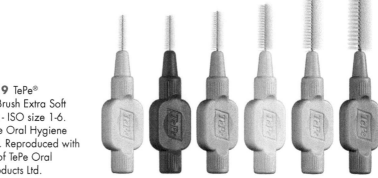

Figure 8.19 TePe® Interdental Brush Extra Soft Mixed Pack - ISO size 1-6. Source: TePe Oral Hygiene Products Ltd. Reproduced with permission of TePe Oral Hygiene Products Ltd.

OTHER DISEASES AND DISORDERS AFFECTING THE ORAL CAVITY

aware of these and consult the patient, relatives, and oncology professionals. They can also recommend:

- Gentle mouth brushing with a very soft brush (e.g. TePe® Special Care Toothbrush, Figure 8.18) and TePe® Extra Soft Interdental Brush (Figure 8.19).
- Using a sonic toothbrush.
- Sucking ice chips.

Prevention

The following measures should be taken to reduce the risk of mouth cancer:

- Cease smoking/chewing tobacco (see Chapter 13).
- Keep within safe alcohol limits (see Chapter 13).
- Maintain a good diet (see Chapter 9).
- Avoid prolonged exposure to strong sunlight and use sunblock on lips.
- Regular dental checks (for early diagnosis).

SQUAMOUS CELL PAPILLOMA

Squamous cell papillomas (Figure 8.20) are formed as a result of an overgrowth of epithelial (skin) cells, which become keratinised and develop folds or fronds. Common sites for occurrence are the lips and palate, but they can occur anywhere in the oral cavity.

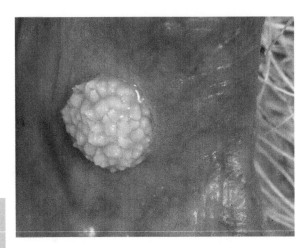

Figure 8.20 Squamous Cell Papilloma Source: Professor M.A.O. Lewis, Cardiff University. Reproduced with permission of Professor M.A.O. Lewis.

Aetiology

Squamous cell papillomas are a result of infection with the human papilloma virus (HPV), and are benign in nature.

Clinical features

Clinical features of a squamous cell papilloma include:

- A few millimetres across in size.
- Irregular in shape – often with finger-like or cauliflower-like projections.
- Usually painless.

Treatment

No treatment is required unless they affect eating or become painful, in which case a simple surgical excision can be performed.

MUCOCELE

A mucocele (Figure 8.21) is a cystic swelling affecting minor salivary glands, usually found on the lower lip or buccal mucosa.

Clinical features

Clinical features of a mucocele include:

- Broad-based swelling, slightly translucent with a blue tinge.
- Mucous-filled cyst.
- Can vary in size, from 1 mm to several centimetres across.

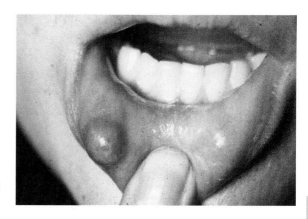

Figure 8.21 Mucocele on the lower lip. Source: [4]. Reproduced with permission of Wiley Blackwell.

Aetiology

Causes of a mucocele include:

- Trauma, which causes the gland duct to rupture and so saliva is unable to escape.
- Patient gives history of a rapid swelling, like a balloon after trauma.

Treatment

Treatment of a mucocele includes:

- Can be self-healing.
- Minor surgical removal.

TORI

Tori (*sing. torus*) are normal bony growths that appear on the lingual side of the mandible in the floor of the mouth (Figure 8.22) and the midline of the palate. *Exostoses* (*sing. exostosis*) describe the formation of new bone (on the surface of bone) and usually form bilaterally.

Although benign, if they become too large, they can restrict tongue movement or alter speech. The dental professional should be aware that they can be a problem when taking impressions or making dental appliances. It is possible to remove them surgically after which they will not grow back. Most patients who have them are unaware as they are part of their normal mouth structure.

BURNS

Burns can occur anywhere on the soft tissues of the oral cavity and can be quite alarming in appearance (Figure 8.23).

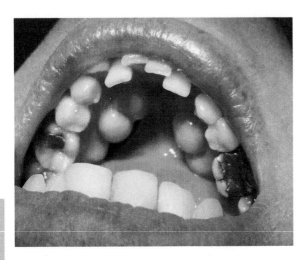

Figure 8.22 Lingual tori.
Source: Alison Chapman.

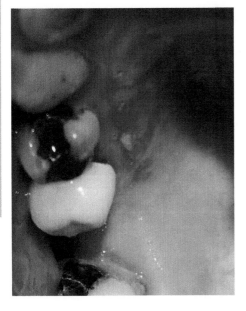

Figure 8.23 Burn on hard palate.
Source: Alison Chapman.

Aetiology

The cause of a burn should become obvious on discussion with the patient. Causes of burns include:

- Heat – such as very hot food (e.g. cheese on a pizza) or liquids.
- Chemical – such as a patient placing an aspirin next to a painful tooth, which burns the tissues as it dissolves.

Clinical features

Clinical features of burns include:

- Red and/or white patches, which may have skin peeling from them.
- Can be any size or shape.
- Pain – can be severe.

Treatment

Treatment of a burn depends on the severity and includes:

- None – often self-heal, or begin to heal within a few days.
- Analgesics.
- Chlorhexidine mouthwash to reduce the chance of secondary infection.
- Ice chips applied to the affected area.

RECREATIONAL DRUG USERS

Recreational drug users (people who regularly take cannabis, heroin, and other drugs not prescribed as part of medical treatment), are particularly prone to oral diseases associated with lowered immunity. OHEs should be aware that patients who repeatedly present with conditions such as NUG, Candida, and herpetic infections could be using recreational drugs (see Chapter 13).

SYSTEMIC DISEASES WITH ORAL IMPLICATIONS

A systemic disease is one that affects the whole body, such as diabetes, epilepsy, lichen planus, acquired immune deficiency syndrome (AIDS), Crohn's disease, colitis, and Sjögren's syndrome. These diseases can present with oral manifestations.

Diabetes

Diabetes is caused by the pancreas failing to produce sufficient insulin (a hormone which converts glucose into energy), and is characterised by persistent hyperglycaemia (high blood sugar level). There are two main forms of this disease: type 1 and type 2 diabetes.

OTHER DISEASES AND DISORDERS AFFECTING THE ORAL CAVITY

Type 1 diabetes

Type 1 diabetes, also known as insulin-dependent diabetes mellitus (IDDM), often begins in childhood or adolescence and the patient usually requires insulin injections from diagnosis. Patients must stick to dietary recommendations or otherwise face potential complications in later life, including eye problems and difficulties with peripheral circulation leading to soft tissue and organ damage.

Type 2 diabetes

Type 2 diabetes, also known as non-insulin-dependent diabetes mellitus (NIDDM), usually begins in later life and may involve a hereditary factor. Patients are often unfit and overweight before the disease develops. It can usually be controlled by diet and tablets, but sometimes insulin injections are required. Complications are similar to those associated with type 1.

Oral implications of diabetes

Oral implications (particularly periodontitis) in both types of diabetes are due to:

- Blood vessel degeneration – vessels are less able to transport an adequate blood supply, which helps repair and maintain tissue.
- Altered collagen metabolism – the body is less able to produce good quality collagen for adequate tissue repair and maintenance.
- Certain types of white blood cells become less attracted to sites of infection, and diabetics are less able to fight infection.

A study by the UCL Eastman Dental Institute (funded by Diabetes UK) has found that treating gum disease can help people with type 2 diabetes manage blood glucose, and may reduce their risk of diabetes-related complications. Gum disease causes inflammation inside the body, and this has been linked to insulin resistance – a key aspect of type 2 diabetes [10].

Patients with epilepsy

Patients with epilepsy may have gingivitis or gingival overgrowth associated with taking anticonvulsant drugs, e.g. phenytoin (see Chapter 3). These patients also require special care in the dental surgery (see Chapter 24).

Lichen planus

Lichen planus (Figure 8.24) is a systemic skin condition that can also affect the mouth. It principally affects the buccal mucosa, but the tongue, lips, and attached gingivae can also be affected. This condition can also be seen elsewhere on the body, appearing as a persistent rash. In rare cases, it can be pre-malignant but not unless changes (such as ulceration and pain) occur. Sometimes there are no oral symptoms, but occasionally they present in the oral cavity and not elsewhere.

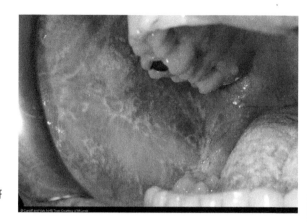

Figure 8.24 Lichen planus
Source: Professor M.A.O.
Lewis, Cardiff University.
Reproduced with permission of
Professor M.A.O. Lewis.

Aetiology

The cause(s) of lichen planus are unknown.

Clinical features

Clinical features of lichen planus include:

- Interlacing network of white striae (striped skin lesions) – commonly seen on the buccal mucosa.
- Red sores – commonly seen on the gingivae (often painless).

Treatment

Treatment of lichen planus includes:

- Gentle oral hygiene instruction. Consider:
  - A soft toothbrush or sonic power brush.
  - Extra soft interdental brushes.
  - Sodium lauryl sulphate (SLS) free toothpaste.
  - Flavourless toothpaste.
- Steroid mouthwash (for acute conditions).
- Avoidance of irritants (e.g. spicy or acidic foods).

Acquired immune deficiency syndrome (AIDS)

Aetiology

AIDS is caused by the human immunodeficiency virus (HIV).

Oral manifestations

Oral signs and symptoms of AIDS include:

- Marginal gingivitis, sometimes severe with ulcers.
- NUG – widespread ulceration (see Chapter 4).

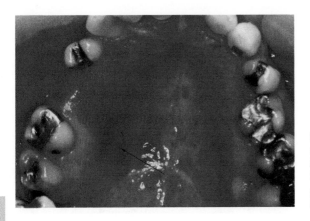

Figure 8.25 Kaposi's sarcoma. Source: Professor M.A.O. Lewis, Cardiff University. Reproduced with permission of Professor M.A.O. Lewis.

- Oral thrush – recurrent and persistent.
- Herpes simplex virus and zoster (shingles).
- Swelling of cervical lymph nodes.
- Kaposi's sarcoma (Figure 8.25) – cancerous tumour in rare, late stage. Painless purple swelling usually on the palate.

Treatment

Treatment of these manifestations includes:

- Systemic drugs and palliative care – keeping the mouth as comfortable and healthy as possible.
- Regular, careful scaling.
- Mouthwashes.
- Antibiotics.

Crohn's disease and colitis

These diseases sometimes present oral manifestations, since in some unfortunate patients the whole of the digestive system, including the mouth, is affected. Patients can show signs of gingivitis and severe ulceration (despite good oral hygiene in many cases).

Sjögren's syndrome *(pronounced show-grins)*

Aetiology

Sjögren's syndrome is an autoimmune disorder identified by its two most common symptoms; dry eyes and dry mouth (xerostomia, see Chapter 7). It is often associated with other autoimmune conditions such as rheumatoid arthritis and lupus.

Clinical features

The mucous membranes and moisture secreting glands of the mouth and eyes are affected resulting in decreased tears and saliva. It is more common in women, and most people are older than 40 at the time of diagnosis.

Treatment

There is no cure, and so treatment is palliative, including:

- Dietary advice to reduce sugar frequency.
- Saliva substitutes and moisturising gels.
- SLS-free toothpaste.
- Frequent sips of water.
- Chewing gum (containing xylitol) to stimulate saliva flow.
- Fluoride mouthwash/high fluoride toothpaste.
- Drugs, such as pilocarpine, to increase saliva flow.
- Stopping smoking and alcohol.

REFERENCES

1. Sanz, M., Herrera, D. & van Winkelhoff, A.J. (2003) The periodontal abscess. In: *Clinical Periodontology and Implant Dentistry* (eds. J. Lindhe, H.T. Karring & N.P. Lang), 4th edn, pp. 260–268. Blackwell Munksgaard, Oxford.
2. Holmstrup, P. & van Steenbergh, D. (2003) Non-plaque induced inflammatory gingival lesions. In: *Clinical Periodontology and Implant Dentistry* (eds. J. Lindhe, H.T. Karring & N.P. Lang), 4th edn, pp. 269–297. Blackwell Munksgaard, Oxford.
3. Lee, S.M.G. & Lee, G.T.R. (2012) Paediatric dentistry. In: *Clinical Textbook of Dental Hygiene and Therapy* (ed. S.L. Noble SL), 2nd edn, pp. 245–247. Wiley Blackwell, Oxford.
4. Farthing, P. (2013) Oral medicine and pathology. *Clinical Textbook of Dental Hygiene and Therapy*. (ed. S.L. Noble SL), 2nd edn, p. 68. Wiley Blackwell, Oxford.
5. Oxford Radcliffe Hospitals NHS Trust (2013) *Burning Mouth Syndrome Information for patients*. Available at: www.uclh.nhs.uk/PandV/PIL/Patient%20information%20 leaflets/Burning%20mouth%20syndrome.pdf [accessed March 25 2019].
6. Cochrane (17 November 2016) *Interventions for treating burning mouth syndrome*. Available at: www.cochrane.org/CD002779/ORAL_interventions-treating-burning-mouth-syndrome [accessed March 25 2019].
7. The Leeds Teaching Hospital NHS Trust (2019) *Burning Mouth Syndrome*. Available at: www.leedsth.nhs.uk/a-z-of-services/oral-and-maxillofacial-surgery/your-condition-and-treatment/burning-mouth-syndrome/ [accessed March 25 2019].
8. The Oral Cancer Foundation (2019) *Oral Cancer Facts*. Available at: www.oralcancerfoundation.org/facts [accessed 29 March 2019].

OTHER DISEASES AND DISORDERS AFFECTING THE ORAL CAVITY

9. Cancer Research UK (2015) *Head and neck cancers statistics*. Available at: www.cancerresearchuk.org/health-professional/cancer-statistics/statistics-by-cancer-type/head-and-neck-cancers#heading-Four [accessed 29 March 2019].

10. Diabetes UK (2018) *Treating gum disease may help manage Type 2 diabetes*. Available at: www.diabetes.org.uk/about_us/news/treating-gum-disease [accessed March 30 2019].

OTHER DISEASES AND DISORDERS AFFECTING THE ORAL CAVITY

Section 3

Oral Disease Prevention

INTRODUCTION

The prevention of oral diseases is now seen as a vital part of dental care for all patients, not just those considered at-risk, and the educator has an important part to play.

This section explores what measures can be taken by both the patient and the dental team in preventing oral diseases through good general health of the oral cavity and whole-body health, which are often linked.

Patients need to be encouraged to take responsibility for their own health, by eating a healthy, balanced diet, reducing sugar and alcohol consumption, giving up smoking, taking regular physical exercise, as well as being advised on fissure sealing and anti-plaque agents.

Chapter 9

Nutrition, diet, and exercise

Learning outcomes

By the end of this chapter you should be able to:

1. Describe what constitutes a healthy, well-balanced diet.
2. Explain *nutrition* and *nutrients*.
3. Detail the effects of dietary deficiencies on oral health.
4. Define *food additives* and *'E' numbers*.
5. Discuss food-labelling laws.
6. Give basic advice and signposting on physical exercise.

INTRODUCTION

One of the most important roles of the oral health educator (OHE) is to advise patients about healthier eating as part of oral and wider general health [1].

In all countries within the UK, the majority of the adult population (aged 18–65) is either classified as being overweight or obese. This is measured using the Body Mass Index (BMI) and calculated by dividing weight by height squared (kg/m^2) [2]:

- Healthy range – with a BMI between 18.5–24.9.
- Overweight – with a BMI between 25–25.9.
- Obese – with a BMI of 30 or greater.

According to The Health Survey for England (2015), approximately 61% of adults are either overweight or obese [2]. Similar figures have been recorded in other surveys for Scotland, Northern Ireland, and Wales [3].

The National Child Measurement Programme (NCMP) has found that approximately 10% of reception age children and 20% of Year 6 children are obese [4].

Basic Guide to Oral Health Education and Promotion, Third Edition.
Alison Chapman and Simon H. Felton.
© 2021 John Wiley & Sons Ltd. Published 2021 by John Wiley & Sons Ltd.
Companion website: www.wiley.com/go/felton/oralhealth

Research from the Global Burden of Disease Study published in the Lancet found that diet is a bigger killer than smoking (particularly diet-related deaths through cardiovascular disease), and is involved in around one in five deaths in the world [5].

ROLE OF THE OHE

Oral health education and promotion has an important role in helping to promote healthy eating and facilitating patients to achieve good general and oral health. Patients will have different dietary demands largely based on their energy needs, yet many people routinely eat more than they need and/or unhealthily.

One of the key health messages that the OHE can give to patients, which is particularly related to the oral cavity as well as general health, is to reduce the amount and frequency of foods and drinks high in salt and added sugar. Such is the importance of reducing sugar frequency intake in the diet and its relationship with the oral cavity in particular, that there is a dedicated chapter on this topic (see Chapter 10).

The OHE should also be able to advise and signpost patients towards achieving a good balanced diet and wellbeing through physical exercise.

A HEALTHY BALANCED DIET (THE EATWELL GUIDE)

Diet refers to the type and amount of food and drink we consume. *The Eatwell Guide* (Figure 9.1) shows the proportions of the different types of food groups we need to eat to have a well-balanced and healthy diet, and reduce the risk of heart disease, stroke, cancer and other conditions, such as type 2 diabetes (see Chapter 8).

The Eatwell Guide applies to most people, except those with special dietary needs who should seek advice from a registered dietician, and children under 2 years old who have different nutritional needs. It recommends that the daily calorific intake for men and women are 2500 and 2000 kcal, respectively.

You should advise patients that they should aim to get this balance of the different types of food groups right each day, but not necessarily for each meal. For some patients, it may be easier to get the balance right over a week. It would be beneficial to download and print copies of The Eatwell Guide to show patients, and consider using as part of a Preventative Dental Unit (PDU) display (see Chapter 17).

NUTRITION, DIET, AND EXERCISE

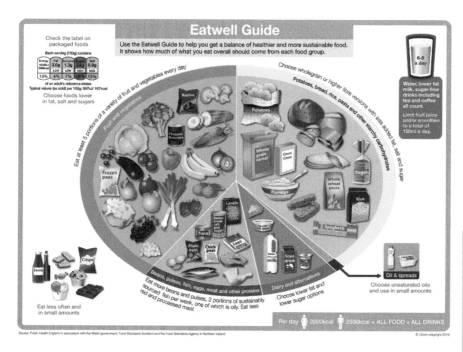

Figure 9.1 The Eatwell Guide. Source: From [6]. ©Crown copyright 2018. Contains public sector information licensed under the Open Government Licence v3.0.

Based on the Eatwell Guide, patients should be advised to eat the following [6]:

- Fruit and vegetables – at least five portions a day (one portion is roughly a handful). A variety of fruit and vegetables is recommended, which can be fresh, frozen, tinned, dried, or juiced. However, fruit juice and smoothies should be limited to 150 ml per day, and are best drunk at mealtimes to reduce caries.
- Meals should be based on starchy carbohydrates – bread, cereals, pasta, rice, and potatoes. Patients should aim for high fibre wholegrain varieties and leave skins on potatoes.
- Dairy/dairy alternatives – an important source of protein and calcium (for bone strength) – choosing lower fat and low sugar options.
- Meat, fish, eggs, beans/pulses – good sources of protein, vitamins, and minerals. Beans and lentils are good alternatives to meat as lower in fat. Eat less red meat and processed meat, and aim for two portions of sustainably sourced fish per week (one being an oily fish like salmon or mackerel, high in unsaturated fat).

NUTRITION, DIET, AND EXERCISE

- Oils and spreads – Choose unsaturated oils and spreads (like olive and vegetable oil), which can lower bad cholesterol. Reduce saturated fats (such as those found in butter and ghee), which can increase bad cholesterol in the blood and contribute to heart disease.
- Less salt and sugar – Choose foods low in salt and sugar. Adults should eat no more than 6 g of salt a day and children even less (6 g of salt is about a teaspoonful) [1]. Much of our salt and sugar in the UK is hidden and comes from ready prepared meals.
- Reduce snacks – Such as cakes, biscuits, chocolate confectionary, pastries, ice cream, and fizzy drinks.
- Drink plenty of water – to keep hydrated. The UK government recommends 6–8 glasses a day (including water, low-fat milk, sugar-free drinks, tea, and coffee).

NUTRITION

Nutrition describes the process by which we absorb and use the food in our diet for energy, growth, and repair of tissue. For our bodies to work efficiently, the following nutritional substances (nutrients) are essential in the correct proportions:

- Carbohydrates.
- Proteins.
- Fats.
- Vitamins.
- Minerals.
- Fibre.
- Water.

Carbohydrates

Carbohydrates should comprise approximately 50% of total daily calorie intake, and provide the biggest source of energy. They are too complex to be absorbed directly by the body and are therefore broken down into smaller units: monosaccharides, disaccharides, and polysaccharides.

The glycaemic index (GI) is a rating that shows how quickly a food containing carbohydrates affects blood sugar (glucose) levels when that food is eaten on its own. High-GI foods (including sugar, potatoes, and white rice) are broken down quickly and cause a rapid increase in blood sugar. Low and medium GI foods (including fruits, vegetables, and wholegrain foods) are broken down more slowly and cause a more gradual rise in blood sugar.

Proteins

Proteins should comprise approximately 10–15% of our daily energy intake, and are broken down into amino acids during digestion and absorbed into the body. As well as providing energy, proteins are bodybuilders, being essential for cell growth and repair.

Proteins are made up of long chains of amino acids, and the chemical properties of these acids determine the biological activity of the protein. Some of these amino acids are nutritionally essential as they cannot be made or stored within the body, and so must come from our diet.

Fats

Foods containing fats should comprise approximately a third of total daily energy intake, and are essential to many body processes, although nutritionists encourage people to study the quantities and balance of different fats consumed to reduce the risks of heart disease and other illness.

Fats keep the body warm, metabolise cholesterol, and act as a reserve source of energy. Saturated fats and unsaturated fats contain the same amount of calories, but, as mentioned, patients should be advised to eat more of the healthy unsaturated fats and cut down on saturated fats.

Vitamins

Vitamins are a group of complex organic substances that occur in minute amounts in foods. Even though they are found in such small amounts, they are essential for our bodies to work properly. They cannot be synthesised by the body in an adequate supply, and are absorbed unchanged from foodstuffs. The absence of certain vitamins in tissues can cause deficiency syndromes.

Vitamin classification

Vitamins are classified according to whether they are fat-soluble or water-soluble. Unsurprisingly, fat-soluble vitamins are found mainly in fatty foods, and while the body needs them, you do not need to eat foods containing them every day because they are stored in the liver and fatty tissues to be used when required.

If patients eat a balanced diet, they should get the vitamins they need, although certain medical conditions and situations (e.g. pregnancy) require supplements and should be prescribed by the doctor. However, taking too many supplements, or for too long, can be harmful to health.

NUTRITION, DIET, AND EXERCISE

Fat-soluble vitamins

Fat-soluble vitamins include:

- Vitamin A – found in fish oils, eggs, milk, green vegetables, and carrots. It protects against infection, influences changes in epithelial cells, and helps eyes see in dim light.
- Vitamin D – found in dairy products, fish and fish oils, and also synthesised from sunlight by the body. It regulates calcium and phosphorus metabolism and helps with the calcification of bones and teeth, protecting against rickets.
- Vitamin E – found in nuts, lettuce, egg yolk, wheat germ, cereals, milk, and butter. Function is not fully understood, but believed to be concerned with preventing muscle waste, and aiding fertility.
- Vitamin K – found in fish, liver, leafy green vegetables, and fruit. It is concerned with blood clotting.

Water-soluble vitamins

Water-soluble vitamins are not stored in the body and so need to be taken more frequently. Some are found in vegetables, and as they are water soluble they can be lost to water on boiling. That is why it is best to steam or grill vegetables rather than boil them.

Water-soluble vitamins include:

- Vitamin B complex – so-called, because there are several types (e.g. B6, B12, folic acid). B vitamins are found in vegetables, starch, seeds, grains and pulses, eggs, fish, and meat. A deficiency can cause anaemia, digestive disorders, skin problems, bleeding gums, and glossitis (see Chapter 8).
- Vitamin C – found in fruit and vegetables. A deficiency can cause scurvy, bone fractures, skin lesions, bleeding gums, and damage to the periodontal ligament.

Minerals

Minerals are absorbed directly from the diet. They are found in minute amounts in most foods, and include:

- Calcium.
- Sodium.
- Potassium.
- Phosphorus.
- Magnesium.
- Iron.

- Chloride.
- Iodine.
- Fluoride.

Minerals are important for:

- Building strong bones and teeth.
- Controlling body fluids.
- Converting food into energy.

Fibre

Fibre only comes from food made from plants (e.g. fruit, vegetables, seeds, and pulses). There are two main types:

- Insoluble fibre. The body cannot digest this type of fibre, so it passes through the gastrointestinal tract, helping other food and waste products move through the tract more easily. Wholegrain bread and breakfast cereals, brown rice, and wholewheat pasta are good sources of this type of fibre.
- Soluble fibre. This type of fibre can be partly digested and may help reduce the amount of cholesterol in the blood. Oats and pulses are good sources.

Water

Water is, of course, essential for life. A human being can survive for several weeks without food, but will die in a few days from dehydration. To stay healthy, it is vital to replace the fluid that is lost when we breathe, sweat, or urinate.

The amount of water an individual requires to prevent dehydration varies depending on a range of factors, including their size, the ambient temperature, and how active they are. But, as mentioned, 6–8 glasses of fluid a day are recommended as a general guide [6].

FOOD ADDITIVES

A food additive (e.g. monosodium glutamate) is a substance not normally consumed as a food by itself, and not normally used as a typical ingredient of food, whether it has nutritive value or not.

NUTRITION, DIET, AND EXERCISE

Food additives are normally non-nutrients (i.e. we do not need them to survive), but they are used to improve flavour, colouring, shelf-life, and convenience in cooking. They often get a bad press, being held responsible for everything from hyperactivity in children to various food allergies. However, their addition to foods is strictly controlled in the EU and EFTA countries under EU food additives legislation, and each permitted additive is given an *'E' number ('E' stands for Europe)*, which signifies that they have been tested and passed for use. This number must be printed on the food label.

Internationally, the Joint FAO/WHO Expert Committee on Food Additives (JECFA) is responsible for evaluating the safety of food additives, and only those deemed safe by JECFA can be used for foods traded between nations.

FOOD LABELLING

Food labelling law is complex, and requirements vary according to food type, and are regulated by EU directives for the UK (at the time of writing). For example, pre-packed foods require a nutritional declaration per 100 g/mL or per portion, including energy value (in kJ and kcal), and the amount (in grams) of carbohydrate, protein, sugars, fat, and salt.

The OHE should be able to provide basic guidance on guided daily amounts (GDAs). Guided daily amount labels (also known as *traffic light labels*) are used on many pre-packaged foods (Figure 9.2). It is a voluntary scheme under the Food Information Regulation. The labelling provides nutritional information on the number of calories, as well as fat, saturated fat, sugar, and salt content. The GDA label also includes colour coding for each of these constituents to signal whether a food is high or low in each. Red is *high*, amber is *medium*, and green is *low*. If a food label is mostly coded green it is therefore a healthier option, amber is ok and can be consumed reasonably frequently but not all the time, while red is a warning that we should be eating these types of food less regularly and in small amounts.

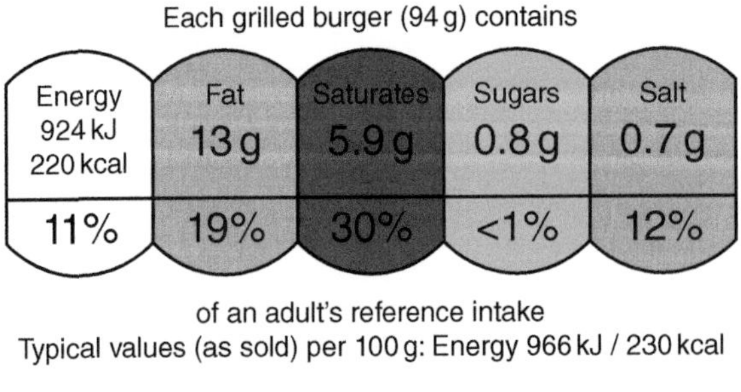

Each grilled burger (94 g) contains

Energy 924 kJ 220 kcal	Fat 13 g	Saturates 5.9 g	Sugars 0.8 g	Salt 0.7 g
11%	19%	30%	<1%	12%

of an adult's reference intake
Typical values (as sold) per 100 g: Energy 966 kJ / 230 kcal

Figure 9.2 Illustration of a Front of Pack (FoP) nutrition label. Source: From [7]. ©Crown copyright 2018. Contains public sector information licensed under the Open Government Licence v3.0.

When giving advice on GDA labels, you must bear in mind that the percentages given are often only for a portion (by weight) of the food, rather than the whole amount of the food.

PHYSICAL EXERCISE AND GENERAL WELLBEING

While it is not the role of the OHE to give advice on physical activity, it is useful to be aware of general recommended activity guidelines in relation to whole body health as a health educator and for when working with other professionals in health promotion; in helping to reduce the risk of heart disease, stroke, cancer and other conditions, such as type 2 diabetes, which can have oral manifestations.

In the UK, the NHS has produced Physical Activity Guidelines for various age groups, which are a good benchmark for the OHE to give basic advice on, or signpost patients towards [8].

Exercise recommendations for adults

The NHS advises that adults should try to be active daily and should do two types of physical activity each week to stay healthy or improve health. Although the recommended amount of exercise for age groups 18–64 and 65 plus is the same, the type of exercise should be tailored according to age (for example a 70-year-old would not be advised to play rugby!).

Adults are recommended to undertake weekly [8]:

- Aerobic exercise, either:
  - 150 minutes of moderate activity, such as cycling/walking/lawn mowing (Figure 9.3), or
  - 75 minutes of vigorous activity, such as running, tennis singles, or football, or
  - A mixture of moderate and vigorous activity amounting to 150 minutes of moderate intensity. (Roughly one minute of vigorous activity provides the same health benefits as two minutes of moderate activity, and so 2 x 30 minute runs and 1 x 30 minutes of brisk walking equates to 150 minutes of moderate activity.)
- Strength exercise:
  - On two or more days a week, working major muscles of the body, including arms, legs, hips, back, abdomen, chest and shoulders, such as yoga, lifting weights, and heavy gardening.

There is evidence that vigorous activity can bring greater health benefits over moderate activity. For a moderate to vigorous workout, patients could try 'Couch to 5K', a 9-week running plan for beginners. Some vigorous activities

NUTRITION, DIET, AND EXERCISE

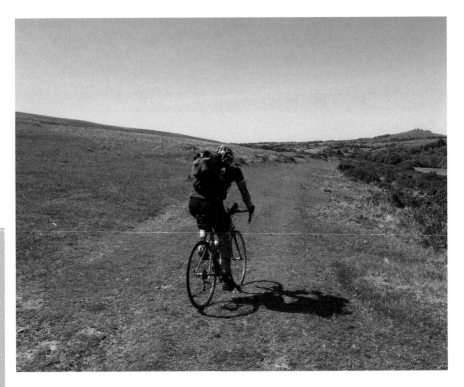

Figure 9.3 Cycling is great exercise. Source: Simon Felton.

count as both an aerobic activity and a muscle-strengthening activity, including netball/basketball, circuit training, and rugby. Strength exercise helps to build and maintain strong bones, regulate blood sugar and blood pressure, and helps maintain a healthy weight.

Exercise recommendations for children

Children under 5 years old

For children (under 5 years), the NHS advises that they are not inactive for long periods when awake, such as being strapped in a buggy or watching TV for too long. They should engage in light activity, such as walking and less energetic play, as well as regular energetic activity, such as running around, riding a bike, swimming and skipping

Children and young people aged 5–18 years old

For children and young people (5–18 year olds) the NHS recommends at least 60 minutes of physical activity every day – from moderate (e.g. cycling, walking, skateboarding) to vigorous activity (e.g. running, swimming, dancing).

On three days a week, activity should involve high intensity activities, including those that strengthen muscle and bone. For children, these activities include skipping, fast running, lifting their own body weight in playground equipment and gymnastics, dance, and football. For young people, activities include aerobics, running, gymnastics, weight training, rugby, and hockey.

Young people should also reduce sedentary time and there are no recommendations on how long a session of vigorous activity should be for this group.

REFERENCES

1. Public Health England and Department of Health (2017) *Delivering better oral health: an evidence-based toolkit for prevention.* Available at: www.gov.uk/government/publications/delivering-better-oral-health-an-evidence-based-toolkit-for-prevention [accessed 30 April 2019].

2. NHS Digital (2015) *The Health Survey for England.* Available at: https://webarchive.nationalarchives.gov.uk/20180307193646/http://digital.nhs.uk/catalogue/PUB22610 [accessed 4 April 2019].

3. House of Commons Library Briefing Paper (Number 3336, 20 March 2018) *Obesity Statistics.* Available at: https://researchbriefings.files.parliament.uk/documents/SN03336/SN03336.pdf [accessed 4 April 2019].

4. NHS Digital (2016) *National Child Measurement Programme - England, 2015-16.* Available at: https://digital.nhs.uk/data-and-information/publications/statistical/national-child-measurement-programme/2015-16-school-year [accessed 4 April 2019].

5. Afshin, A., Sur, P., Fay, K. & Cornaby, L. (2019) (Global Burden of Disease Study 2017 Diet Collaborators). Health effects of dietary risks in 195 countries, 1990–2017: a systematic analysis for the Global Burden of Disease Study 2017. *The Lancet,* 393(10184), 1958–1972.

6. Public Health England (2018) *The Eatwell Guide – A Balanced Diet.* Available at: https://assets.publishing.service.gov.uk/government/uploads/system/uploads/attachment_data/file/742750/Eatwell_Guide_booklet_2018v4.pdf [accessed 4 April 2019].

7. Department of Health (June 2013) *Guide to creating a front of pack (FoP) nutrition label for pre-packed products sold through retail outlets.* Available at: https://assets.publishing.service.gov.uk/government/uploads/system/uploads/attachment_data/file/566251/FoP_Nutrition_labelling_UK_guidance.pdf [accessed 22 January 2020].

8. NHS (10/07/2018) *Exercise.* Available at: www.nhs.uk/live-well/exercise/physical-activity-guidelines-children-under-five-years/ [accessed 4 April 2019].

Chapter 10

Sugars in the diet

Learning outcomes

By the end of this chapter you will be able to:

1. Differentiate between *intrinsic, free,* and *milk* sugars, and list the food groups in which they are found.
2. Define SACN and list its recommendations on *free sugar* consumption.
3. Give advice to patients on sugar consumption – quantity and frequency.
4. Define *hidden sugars,* and list common sugars found on food labels.
5. Define *artificial sweeteners,* and distinguish between *bulk* and *intensive* sweeteners, stating the sources and uses of each.

INTRODUCTION

The overconsumption of sugar in its various forms has long been associated with the development of caries (see Chapter 5). It has also been identified as a major factor in obesity (see Chapter 9), and the growth of other non-communicable diseases (NCDs), particularly type 2 diabetes, cardiovascular disease (CVD), and cancer. Furthermore, it has been linked to childhood behavioural problems, and detrimental health effects during weaning.

Of particular concern is the consumption of free sugars (see following Classification of sugars), which are the sugars most responsible for dental caries. According to the World Health Organization (WHO), people who have a higher intake of free sugars have more dental caries [1].

UK CONSUMPTION

In the UK, the current average intake of free sugars is at least twice the 5% recommendation for adults and children (and three times the recommendation in 11-18 year olds); the main sources being sweetened drinks and cereals, confectionery, table sugar, and fruit juices [2].

However, there is some good news. In the UK, surveys between 2008/09 and 2016/17 have shown a downward trend in the consumption of sugar-sweetened soft drinks in all age groups [2]. Furthermore, from the 6th April 2018, the UK government introduced the Soft Drinks Industry Levy, also known as the *Sugar Tax*, to combat childhood obesity (which dental professionals also hope will positively impact oral health). Those who don't reformulate will pay the levy, which will go towards schools' sports facilities and equipment, and healthy school breakfast clubs [3].

But more needs to be done at policy level and in educating individual patients to help them take responsibility, and that's where the OHE comes in; educating the patient on types of sugars and recommendations to help prevent or manage conditions associated with overconsumption.

CLASSIFICATION OF SUGARS

Sugars can be classified into three groups:

1. Free sugars.
2. Intrinsic sugars.
3. Milk sugars.

Free sugars

In 2015, The Scientific Advisory Committee on Nutrition (SACN) recommended that a new definition of *free sugars* should replace the previous term *non-milk extrinsic sugars* (NMES), and has subsequently been adopted by WHO [4]. The SACN advises Public Health England (PHE) and other UK government organisations on nutrition and related health matters, and replaced the Committee on Medical Aspects of Food and Nutrition Policy (COMA).

Free sugars, which include monosaccharides (e.g. glucose and fructose), and disaccharides (e.g. sucrose, maltose), are those sugars [4]:

- Added by the manufacturer, cook, or consumer – including processed foods, such as confectionery, soft drinks, biscuits, and cakes.

SUGARS IN THE DIET

- Naturally present – in unsweetened fruit and vegetable juices, honey, syrup, purees and pastes, and raw sugar (white, brown, muscovado, and cane).
- In drinks (other than from dairy sources), including alcohol.

SACN free sugar recommendations

SACN recommends that [4]:

- The average intake of free sugars, across the UK population (from 2 years old), should not exceed 5% of total dietary energy intake.
- The consumption of sugar-sweetened drinks should be minimised in children and adults.
- The term *free sugars* should be adopted in the UK to describe the types of sugars that need to be consumed in smaller amounts.

These recommendations are designed to not only help improve dental health, but also reduce obesity. For those maintaining a healthy body weight, SACN advises that free sugars should be replaced by other carbohydrate sources, including starches, fruit sugars, and lactose in milk/milk products.

WHO Public Health Recommendations

On a global level, WHO has also published its public health solutions for addressing caries through policy, which includes promotional measures to reduce free sugar consumption, including [1]:

- Clear nutritional labeling.
- Improving the food environment in public institutions (e.g. schools, hospitals, work).
- Increasing awareness/access to safe, clean drinking water.

Intrinsic sugars

Intrinsic sugars are found in the cell walls of whole fruits and vegetables. They also include fructose, glucose, and sucrose (which, confusingly also come in free sugar form), but they do not begin to break down in the mouth (unlike say fructose in fruit juice), and are therefore generally less cariogenic than their free sugar form.

Intrinsic sugars also include processed (dried, stewed, canned, and frozen) fruits, and vegetables. It is recommended that these foods should be limited to mealtimes owing to their potential cariogenic effect on teeth. It must be noted that intrinsic sugars found within the cell wall of fresh fruit and vegetables are less cariogenic than those found in dried, stewed, or canned fruit and vegetables as they do not break down in the mouth.

Milk sugars

Milk sugars (lactose and galactose) occur naturally in milk and dairy products, such as yoghurt and cheese. They are regarded as less cariogenic than free sugars because they are accompanied by other essential nutrients (e.g. calcium), which counteract potential damage to teeth.

OHE ADVICE TO PATIENTS ON SUGAR CONSUMPTION

OHEs should be able to advise patients on the following topics in order to reduce their intake of sugars.

Reduce daily sugar consumption

Patients should be advised to reduce their daily consumption of sugar, if they have not done so already. In 2015, Public Health England (PHE) published their recommended intake of sugars, to be no more than [5]:

- 19 g per day (five sugar cubes) for 4–6 year olds.
- 24 g per day (six sugar cubes) for 6–10 year olds.
- 30 g per day (seven sugar cubes for 11 and over).

It must be noted that this sugar may be *hidden* and difficult to spot (see following text), or added to foods and drinks themselves. The latter can be a hard habit to break for some, particularly when started in childhood. OHEs should advise pregnant women and parents of young children, in particular, that adding sugar to food can contribute to obesity, caries, and behavioural disorders.

Identify hidden sugars (read the label)

Many people still associate sugar with white refined sucrose (table sugar), although public awareness is improving with moves towards healthier eating. It is important to be able to identify hidden sugars (e.g. glucose, fructose, dextrose, maltose, lactose and molasses), and advise patients to look for them on food labels (Figure 10.1).

Reduce frequency of sugar intake

The dental profession has been aware for over half a century that the frequency of sugar intake is far more significant in the development of caries than the amount consumed at any given time (see Chapter 5), and OHEs need to reenforce this message.

SUGARS IN THE DIET

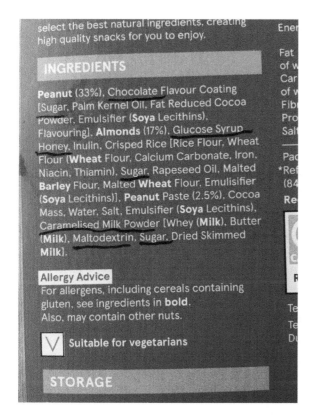

Ener

Fat
of w
Car
of w
Fib
Pro
Sal

Pac
*Re
(84

Re

R

Te
Te
Di

INGREDIENTS

Peanut (33%), Chocolate Flavour Coating
[Sugar, Palm Kernel Oil, Fat Reduced Cocoa
Powder, Emulsifier (**Soya** Lecithins),
Flavouring]. **Almonds** (17%), Glucose Syrup,
Honey, Inulin, Crisped Rice [Rice Flour, **Wheat**
Flour (**Wheat** Flour, Calcium Carbonate, Iron,
Niacin, Thiamin), Sugar, Rapeseed Oil, Malted
Barley Flour, Malted **Wheat** Flour, Emulsifier
(**Soya** Lecithins)], **Peanut** Paste (2.5%), Cocoa
Mass, Water, Salt, Emulsifier (**Soya** Lecithins),
Caramelised Milk Powder [Whey (**Milk**), Butter
(**Milk**), Maltodextrin, Sugar, Dried Skimmed
Milk].

Allergy Advice
For allergens, including cereals containing
gluten, see ingredients in **bold**.
Also, may contain other nuts.

☑ **Suitable for vegetarians**

STORAGE

Figure 10.1 Hidden sugars
(granola health bar). Source:
Alison Chapman.

Sugary foods are best taken during mealtimes, when salivary flow is good, while bedtime is a particularly bad time to consume sugar as the salivary flow rate slows during sleep.

Patients will often ask, and be surprised by, the amounts of sugar in different foods and drinks. It is therefore helpful to be able to give an information sheet, setting out these amounts (5 grams of sugar is roughly 1 teaspoon). When setting up a PDU, producing an exhibition, display or delivering a talk, points about reducing sugar consumption can be emphasised by setting out a table of common snacks and putting sugar lumps or small bowls of sugar beside each to show the amount in each snack or drink (see Chapters 16, 17, 18).

Reduce unhealthy snacks

Patients should reduce all snacks, particularly those containing sugar (and especially free sugars). It is important to give the same advice as other health professionals, such as dieticians and health visitors, who are concerned with healthy eating and obesity (see Chapter 9).

Potentially cariogenic snacks include:

- Sugary soft drinks.
- Sweets and chocolate confectionery.
- Cakes, biscuits, buns, pastries.
- Fruit juices and smoothies.
- Milk-based drinks with added sugar.
- Dried fruits and fruit bars.

Find healthy alternatives

In the past, the dental profession has suggested that plain crisps, peanuts, and cheese were tooth-friendly alternatives to sweets, biscuits, and confectionery. When reading labels, it can be seen that some nut snacks and flavoured crisps contain hidden sugars, and this should be pointed out to patients. OHEs must also be aware that patients may be told by other health professionals to avoid these foods for other health reasons.

Patients should aim to replace snacks high in sugar and saturated fat with healthier alternatives, for example:

- Unsalted mixed nuts (mindful of nut allergies) and seeds.
- Fresh fruit and chopped vegetables (e.g. carrots and pepper).
- Rice cakes (plain).
- Wholegrain and wholemeal products.

Advice must also be balanced by awareness that people (particularly school-children and adolescents), require frequent intakes of carbohydrates to sustain energy, while other groups need less calories (through snacking).

Sugar-free medicines

Patients should be advised to choose sugar-free medicines wherever possible, such as liquid paracetamol and ibuprofen suspensions for children, whether they are off-the-shelf, over-the-counter, or prescribed by their GP.

Products not containing fructose, glucose, or sucrose can be called *sugar-free* on labels. Those containing hydrogenated glucose syrup, lycasin, maltitol, sorbitol, or xylitol are also listed as sugar-free, as considered non-cariogenic. Artificial sweeteners are also listed as sugar-free [6].

Patients on long-term medication for conditions (such as analgesia pain relief, epilepsy, infections) that are not available sugar-free, should be advised to take it at mealtimes (unless this contradicts prescription/product guidelines on taking medicines with an empty stomach). If taking medication in the morning or nighttime, recommend that patients brush their teeth afterwards.

Consider using sugar substitutes

See the text that follows.

SUGAR SUBSTITUTES

The use of artificial sweeteners is increasing as the public becomes more diet conscious, since their low calorific value means that they are virtually non-cariogenic and non-fattening. Sweeteners can be of synthetic or natural origin such as xylitol, which is a non-cariogenic plant extract (see later in chapter).

European Union (EU) permitted sweeteners in the UK fall into two groups: bulk sweeteners and intense sweeteners (identified by *E* numbers on food labels). Many people are concerned about the safety of sugar substitutes, as the public becomes more informed about food additives.

In 1995 the European Economic Community (now the EU) directed:

- The justification of sweeteners in energy-reduced, non-cariogenic food-stuffs, and food without sugars.
- The extension of the numbers of sweeteners used in the UK, ruling that maximum intake levels should be stated on labels.
- Sweeteners may not be used in foods intended for infants and young children.
- Warning labels must be used.
- Sugars must be indicated in the list of ingredients.

Bulk sweeteners

Bulk sweeteners replace sugar weight for weight, look like sugar, and are used in foods where bulk is needed (e.g. in cooking, for diabetics, and in medicines). They can supply similar energy levels as sucrose, and are equally, or slightly less, sweet. They are not readily used by oral bacteria, and do not cause acid attacks unless they are used in conjunction with extrinsic sugars.

The main bulk sweeteners used in the United Kingdom are:

- Sorbitol (E420).
- Mannitol (E421).
- Isomalt (E953).
- Malitol (E965).
- Lactitol (E966).
- Hydrogenated glucose syrup.
- Xylitol (E967) – particularly important since it is non-cariogenic (see following text).

SUGARS IN THE DIET

Xylitol (E967)

Xylitol is a naturally occurring sugar used as a substitute for sucrose (being of similar sweetness). It can be produced from birch trees and is also found in plums, strawberries, raspberries, and rowanberries.

Xylitol contains around a third less calories than sucrose, and has a lesser effect on blood sugar levels and insulin than table sugar (as it is not readily absorbed into the bloodstream). It can therefore be considered as a good alternative to sugar for those seeking to lose weight and for diabetics, although it is recommended patients consult their GP.

Xylitol is commonly used in:

- Chewing gum.
- Mints.
- Medicines.
- Toothpastes.

Research has also shown that xylitol can benefit oral health. Not only does it not cause caries, but it can actually be used in its prevention, as it is thought to help raise the pH of the mouth to a more alkaline state, inhibiting the growth of *Strep. mutans* – the primary bacterium associated with dental caries, as well as stimulating the flow of saliva.

A study in Finland concluded that regular maternal use of the plant extract in the form of chewing gum resulted in a reduction in *mutans streptococci* colonisation in the teeth of 2-year-old children compared with teeth in children whose mothers received fluoride or chlorhexidine varnish treatment. In 5-year-old children, dentinal caries in the xylitol group was reduced by about 70% compared with that in the fluoride or chlorhexidine group [7].

Furthermore, a systematic review of primary xylitol research by the highly regarded Cochrane Network, entitled, *Xylitol-containing products for preventing dental caries in children and adults*, also found evidence that products containing both fluoride and xylitol had a greater effect in preventing caries [8].

However, xylitol can have a laxative effect, so care should be taken when advising its regular use. It should also be recommended that the best way to prevent and manage caries is to avoid excessive and frequent consumption of sugars and sweeteners, and aim for a balanced diet (see Chapter 9).

Xylitol can also be toxic to dogs and can prove fatal if ingested. Dogs have even been poisoned by treading on chewing gum and licking their paws. If a dog is thought to have consumed xylitol, the owner should take it to the vet immediately [9].

Intense sweeteners

Intense sweeteners have no nutritional value, no bulk, and no calories. They are usually manufactured in the form of minute pellets, are up to 300 times sweeter than sucrose and, like bulk sweeteners, are not a substrate for oral bacteria.

The main intense sweeteners used in the UK are used to sweeten tea and coffee, and are also popular with dieters:

- Acesulfame K (E950).
- Aspartame (E951).
- Saccharin (E954).
- Thaumatin (E957).

REFERENCES

1. World Health Organization (2017) *Sugars and dental caries – WHO Technical Information Note.* Available at: www.who.int/oral_health/publications/sugars-dental-caries-keyfacts/en/ [accessed 20 March 2019].
2. Public Health England (2019) *National Diet and Nutrition Survey.* Available at: www.gov.uk/government/statistics/ndns-time-trend-and-income-analyses-for-years-1-to-9 [accessed 20 March 2019].
3. Gov.UK (2018) *Soft Drinks Industry Levy comes into effect.* Available at: www.gov.uk/government/news/soft-drinks-industry-levy-comes-into-effect [accessed 29 April 2019].
4. The Scientific Advisory Committee (2015) *Carbohydrates and Health.* Available at: www.gov.uk/government/publications/sacn-carbohydrates-and-health-report [accessed 29 April 2019].
5. Public Health England (2015) *Sugar reduction: from evidence into action.* Available at: www.gov.uk/government/publications/sugar-reduction-from-evidence-into-action [accessed 3 May 2019].
6. Public Health England and Department of Health (2017). *Delivering better oral health: an evidence-based toolkit for prevention.* Available at: www.gov.uk/government/publications/delivering-better-oral-health-an-evidence-based-toolkit-for-prevention [accessed 30 April 2019].
7. Isokangas, P.R., Soderling, E., Pienihakkinen, K.R. & Alanen, P. (2000) Occurrence of dental decay in children after maternal consumption of xylitol chewing gum: a follow-up from 0 to 5 years of age. *Journal of Dental Research*, 79(11), 1885–1889.
8. Cochrane (2015) *The impact of Cochrane evidence on xylitol for preventing caries.* Available at: www.cochrane.org/news/impact-cochrane-evidence-xylitol-preventing-caries [accessed 29 April 2019].
9. Blue Cross for Pets (2018) *Xylitol poisoning in dogs.* Available at: www.bluecross.org.uk/pet-advice/xylitol-poisoning-dogs [accessed 29 April 2019].

Chapter 11
Fluoride

Learning outcomes

By the end of this chapter you should be able to:

1. Define *fluoride,* state where it is found, and how it works.
2. Differentiate between the *systemic* and *topical* administration of fluoride.
3. List the benefits of fluoride.
4. Define *fluorosis* and its treatment.
5. Give advice on dental products containing fluoride.

WHAT IS FLUORIDE?

Fluoride is a naturally occurring mineral, and is a compound of the element fluorine.

Facts about fluoride

Here are some facts about fluoride:

- It is found in water, soil, rock, air, plants, and food (e.g. fish, tea, and beer).
- It's main function in the body is in the mineralisation of bones and teeth.
- It is readily absorbed from the stomach and rapidly excreted via the kidneys, mostly in urine, and also through sweat and faeces. Traces can be found in hair, tears, breast milk, and saliva.
- Topical fluoride is applied directly to teeth.
- Systemic fluoride is ingested into the body through water or other supplements.
- Calcium fluoride is the form that often occurs naturally in water supplies.

Basic Guide to Oral Health Education and Promotion, Third Edition.
Alison Chapman and Simon H. Felton.
© 2021 John Wiley & Sons Ltd. Published 2021 by John Wiley & Sons Ltd.
Companion website: www.wiley.com/go/felton/oralhealth

- Sodium fluoride is the form used to artificially raise levels in drinking water.
- The amount of fluoride found naturally in water varies from area to area.
- The fluoridation of water is the adjustment, either up or down, of the amount of fluoride in water supplies to an optimum of (1 ppm). The maximum permitted amount of fluoride in drinking water in the UK is 1.5 mg/l (1.5 ppm).
- Evidence shows that fluoride is effective in the prevention of tooth decay (caries).

History of fluoride

It is useful for oral health educators (OHEs) and other health professionals to know a little about the history of fluoride.

1892 (UK)
Sir James Crichton Browne was the first dentist recorded to remark upon the possible connection between fluoride and the incidence of caries [1].

1901 (Colorado Springs, USA)
Dr F. McKay observed 'mottled enamel' in patients, characterised by minute white, yellow or brown spots scattered over tooth surfaces. In certain American states, a relationship between tooth staining and the presence of naturally occurring fluoride in water was observed [2].

1930s (USA)
McKay and Black associated the mottled effect of enamel and low incidence of caries with high levels of fluoride in drinking water [2]. The term *dental fluorosis* was applied to the condition of intrinsic staining caused by fluoride ingestion at over 2 ppm during tooth formation.

Dr H. Trendley-Dean carried out research in South Dakota, Wisconsin, and Colorado. He found that the severity of tooth mottling was affected by the concentration of fluoride in the water, and that a near-maximum reduction in caries occurred when water contained 1 ppm of fluoride [1]. He therefore deduced that 1 ppm was the optimum level to prevent tooth decay in drinking water.

1945 (Michigan, USA)
Sodium fluoride was added to drinking water in Grand Rapids (Michigan), and resulted in a 50% reduction in caries incidence [1].

1955 (UK)
Kilmarnock, Watford and part of Anglesey had 1 ppm fluoride added to the drinking water. After 5 years, a 50% reduction in caries was found [1]. However,

FLUORIDE

local opposition in Kilmarnock halted fluoridated water, and the caries rate rose steadily to previous levels.

1964 (UK)

In 1964, water in the West Midlands and Newcastle was fluoridated.

1978 (UK)

Strathclyde decided to fluoridate its water supply, but this was opposed (partly on the grounds that it could cause cancer), and in a famous case the High Court of Scotland ruled that although water fluoridation was safe and effective, due to a legal technicality, Lord Jauncy found in favour of the opponent [3].

1985 (UK)

The Strathclyde case led to the establishment of a committee, led by Professor Knox, to investigate the possible harmful effects of fluoride. *The Knox Report*, published in 1985, found no evidence that fluoride, when added to water, causes cancer [4].

2000 (UK)

A systematic review (*The York Review*, carried out by the University of York) was commissioned by the chief medical officer of the Department of Health, who requested, *'an up-to-date expert scientific review of fluoride and health'*.

The main conclusions of this review were:

- Fluoride reduces the prevalence of caries.
- A beneficial effect was still evident in nine studies conducted after 1974 (when fluoride was first added to toothpaste).
- Evidence from 15 studies showed that water fluoridation reduces inequalities in dental health across social classes in 5–12 year olds, using the decayed, missing, filled teeth (dmft/DMFT) index (see Chapter 29).
- The prevalence of dental fluorosis increases with the concentration of fluoride in the water.
- No association was found between fluoridated water and bone fractures or bone development problems (29 studies).
- No association was found between water fluoridation and bone, thyroid, and all other cancers (26 studies).

The authors of the review were surprised that, given the level of interest surrounding the issue of public water fluoridation, little high-quality research had been undertaken. They concluded that any future research into the safety and efficacy of water fluoridation should be carried out with appropriate research methods to improve the quality of the existing evidence base [5].

FLUORIDE

2005 (UK)

The British Dental Association (BDA), together with the British Medical Association (BMA) and the British Fluoridation Society, responded to a Primary Care Trust survey of patients in 2005 by asking the House of Lords to amend a bill on the fluoridation of water supplies which was going through Parliament. This was passed in July 2005, allowing the fluoridation of water supplies by local health authorities in England in response to public demand.

2006 (Global)

A World Health Organization (WHO) report found that there was no evidence to suggest that fluoridated water poses a health risk, except in areas with naturally occurring high levels of fluoride in ground water [6]. They also found that caries to be a major public health problem in most high income countries: *'affecting 60-90% of schoolchildren and the vast majority of adults'*.

WHO also concluded that: *'across the world the most important approaches to the effective use of fluorides are automatic fluoridation through water, salt or milk, and self-applied fluoride through use of affordable fluoridated toothpaste'* [7–9].

2012 (UK)

In the UK, the Department of Health continues to be responsible for national policy on fluoridation and the decision to fluoridate a water supply is currently made by Strategic Health Authorities who must carry out a public consultation exercise before deciding whether to fluoridate, then instruct a water company to do so if deemed necessary.

2014 (UK)

Under the Water Industry Act 1991, Public Health England (PHE) has a duty to monitor the effects of fluoride on people living in areas covered by water fluoridation schemes, with a duty to report every four years on behalf of the Secretary of State for Health and Social Care. Their first report was in 2014, which concluded that water fluoridation is an effective and safe public health measure [10].

2015 (UK)

In 2015, a Cochrane Review entitled, *Water fluoridation for the prevention of dental caries, 'evaluated the effects of fluoride in water (added fluoride or naturally occurring) on the prevention of tooth decay and markings on the teeth (fluorosis)'*.

The review found that [11]:

- Water fluoridation is effective at reducing levels of tooth decay in children; the introduction of fluoridation resulted in children having 35% fewer decayed, missing, and filled deciduous teeth, and 26% fewer decayed, missing, and filled permanent teeth.

FLUORIDE

- A fluoride level of 0.7 ppm brings a 12% chance of people having fluorosis that may cause concern about how their teeth look.

However, it must be noted that the results are based on old studies, many of which took place before the introduction of fluoridated toothpaste.

2016 (UK)

The *Code of Practice on the Technical Aspects of Fluoridation of Water Supplies* was published, and set out principles to be followed by water undertakers and licensed suppliers operating fluoridation schemes and safe design and operation of fluoridation installations in England and Wales.

The code ensures [12]:

- Fluoride concentrations in water supplies do not exceed the prescribed concentration of 1.5 mg/l.
- Avoiding over-dosing of fluoridation chemicals.

2018 (UK)

PHE published its second report: *Water fluoridation: health monitoring in England 2018.*

Professor John Newton, Director of Health Improvement at PHE, commented:

'The evidence in this report shows water fluoridation is a safe and effective method to reduce tooth decay, especially among deprived communities. We would encourage local authorities to consider this evidence carefully when deciding on their plans to improve dental health in their areas' [10].

The report found that [10]:

- 5 year olds in areas with water fluoridation schemes were much less likely to experience tooth decay than in areas without schemes.
- The chances of having decayed tooth/teeth extracted in hospital were much lower in areas with water fluoridation.
- Children from all areas benefited from fluoridation, but children from deprived areas benefited most.
- Dental fluorosis, affecting the appearance of teeth, was seen in 10% of children/young people examined in two fluoridated cities.
- Taken alongside wider research, the results do not provide convincing evidence of higher rates of hip fractures, Down's syndrome, kidney stones, bladder cancer, or osteosarcoma (a cancer of the bone) due to fluoridation schemes.

How fluoride works

Fluoride reduces the incidence of caries in the following ways:

- In the developing tooth, calcium hydroxyapatite in enamel is replaced by calcium fluorapatite which withstands a lower pH of 4.5 rather than the normal 5.5. Teeth that erupt with shallower pits and fissures when systemic fluoride is given are more resistant to acid attacks (see Chapter 5).

- Topical fluoride plays a part in ionic exchange, acting as a catalyst, and helping return more acid-resistant crystals to the tooth.
- Fluoride blocks the enzyme systems of plaque bacteria, inhibiting their ability to turn sugars into acids.
- Fluoride has also been shown to remineralise early carious lesions when used topically.

Sources of fluoride

Fluoride can be obtained from water, toothpaste, mouthwash, varnish, tablets and drops, fluoridated milk, and salt.

Water

In the United States over 200 million people drink fluoridated water (added or naturally occurring) [6].

However, approximately 10% of England's population currently receives a water supply which is either naturally or artificially adjusted to the optimum level of 1 mg/l [10].

Regions in England where fluoridation schemes are in place, include parts of (Figure 11.1):

- Eastern England.
- East Midlands.
- North East.
- West Midlands.
- Yorkshire and Humber.

Benefits of water fluoridation

Benefits of water fluoridation include:

- At a concentration of 1 mg/l (1 ppm), fluoridation negates the risk of enamel fluorosis and can reduce caries by 50% (with no patient effort and negligible cost) [1].
- Reduction in caries rate lasts throughout life since the hydroxyapatite of tooth enamel has been replaced by fluorapatite in the developing tooth (fluorapatite is more resistant to acid attacks).
- Economic – it is less expensive to fluoridate water than to fill teeth and treat patients (poor children's oral health is the most common reason for a child to be admitted to hospital in the UK) [6].
- Improves dental health of all who live in a fluoridated area.

For example, in the UK, the beneficial effects of naturally occurring fluoride have been shown by comparing North and South Shields. North Shields

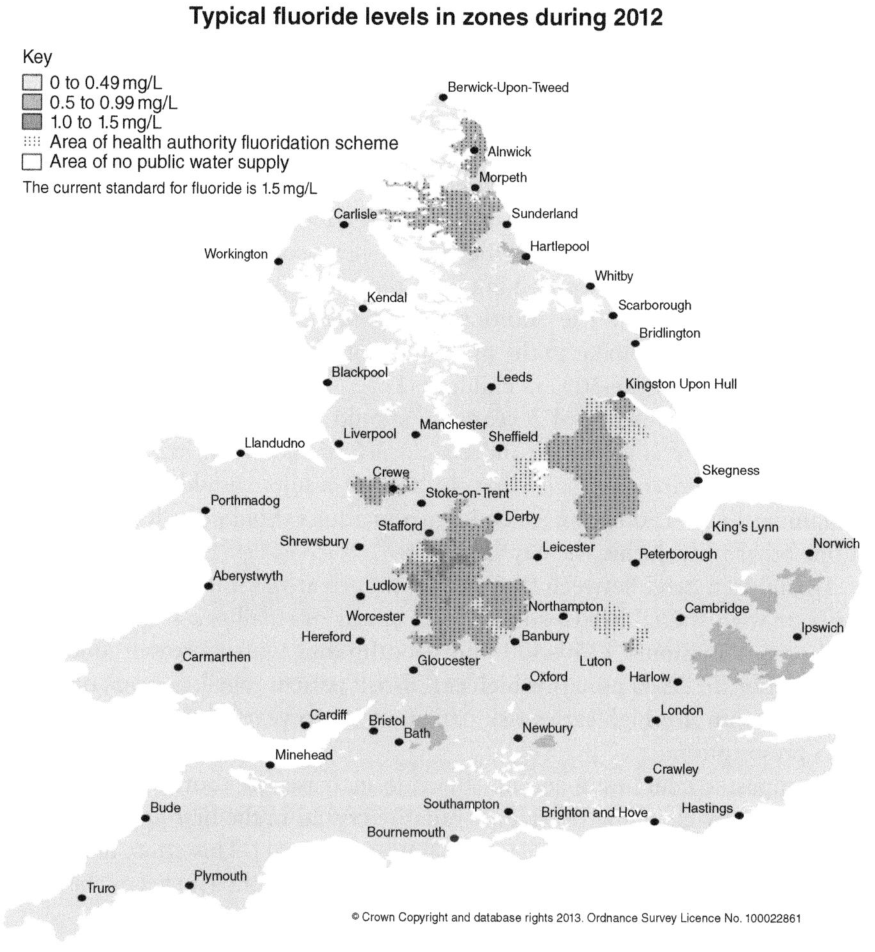

Typical fluoride levels in zones during 2012

Key

☐ 0 to 0.49 mg/L
▨ 0.5 to 0.99 mg/L
▧ 1.0 to 1.5 mg/L
▦ Area of health authority fluoridation scheme
☐ Area of no public water supply

The current standard for fluoride is 1.5 mg/L

Berwick-Upon-Tweed
Alnwick
Morpeth
Carlisle
Sunderland
Workington
Hartlepool
Whitby
Kendal
Scarborough
Bridlington
Blackpool
Leeds
Kingston Upon Hull
Llandudno
Liverpool
Manchester
Sheffield
Crewe
Skegness
Porthmadog
Stoke-on-Trent
Stafford
Derby
King's Lynn
Shrewsbury
Leicester
Norwich
Aberystwyth
Peterborough
Ludlow
Worcester
Northampton
Cambridge
Hereford
Banbury
Ipswich
Carmarthen
Gloucester
Luton
Oxford
Harlow
Cardiff
Bristol
London
Bath
Newbury
Minehead
Crawley
Bude
Southampton
Brighton and Hove
Hastings
Bournemouth
Truro
Plymouth

© Crown Copyright and database rights 2013. Ordnance Survey Licence No. 100022861

Figure 11.1 Typical fluoride levels in zones during 2012. Source: From [13]. ©Crown copyright 2018. Contains public sector information licensed under the Open Government Licence v3.0.

has less than 0.25 ppm fluoride in its water, while South Shields has up to 2 ppm fluoride. In a study, decayed, missing, filled (DMF) index (see Chapter 29) showed that South Shields had almost half the caries rate of North Shields [1].

Opposition to water fluoridation

Despite the clear evidence of the safe and effective use of water fluoridation (at optimum levels) in the prevention of caries, there remains opposition to water fluoridation, with detractors arguing that it is a form of mass medication depriving freedom of choice, can cause fluorosis, and that it should be derived from topical means only.

Toothpastes

Most toothpastes in the UK contain a fluoride compound; either sodium monofluorophosphate, sodium fluoride, or both, and at least one containing a stabilised stannous fluoride [1]. Non-prescription toothpastes contain no more than 1500 ppm of fluoride, and patients should be encouraged to spit after brushing and not rinse toothpaste away.

There is evidence that toothpastes containing higher concentrations of fluoride are more effective at controlling caries when used regularly, and low fluoride toothpastes (those containing less than 1,000ppm) are ineffective at controlling caries [14]. The addition of fluoride to toothpaste has been the biggest single development in the prevention of dental caries, causing a reduction in incidence by 20–30% in children [1].

Children up to the age of 3 years old should use a smear of toothpaste (a thin film of paste covering no more than 3/4 of the brush head) containing 1000 ppm. Children over 3 years old and all adults should use toothpaste containing 1350–1500 ppm. All children and adults should brush at night, and at one other time during the day [14].

All children aged between 0–6 years who are at-risk (i.e. likely to develop caries or with special needs) should use a smear or small *pea-sized* amount of toothpaste containing 1350–500 ppm. Toothpastes with a greater concentration of fluoride: 2800 ppm (for high caries-risk patients aged 10 years or over), and 5000 ppm (for high caries-risk patients over 16 years old) are available on NHS prescription.

Toothpastes containing sodium fluoride increase the tooth's resistance to acid attacks by changing the hydroxyapatite crystal in the first few microns to fluorapatite so that the tooth can withstand a lower pH. This effect diminishes with time after use, and so regular use of a fluoride toothpaste keeps this at an optimal level.

Mouthwash

Mouthwashes containing fluoride can be used daily (0.05% sodium fluoride solution), or weekly (0.2% solution). Daily use is most effective for dentine hypersensitivity and high caries-risk patients. These mouthwashes are also often recommended for patients undertaking fixed appliance therapy.

Mouthwash should be used at a different time from toothbrushing to maximise the topical effect (e.g. after lunch or when return from school/work). Sodium fluoride mouthwash can be recommended for 'at risk' children between 6–10 years old (0.05% daily or 0.2% weekly).

Fluoride varnish

Fluoride varnish is one of the best options for the application of topical fluoride to teeth (regardless of fluoride levels in water), in caries prevention, hypersensitivity, and especially for at-risk children over three years old. It should be used twice yearly, when required as a professional intervention [14]. However, its use is contraindicated in patients with ulcerative gingivitis and stomatitis or in children with a history of asthma.

Systemic reviews have concluded that applications twice yearly or more can produce a mean reduction in caries increment of 37% in the primary dentition and 43% in the permanent dentition, and that it can help stop growth and development of existing lesions on the smooth surfaces of primary teeth and roots of permanent teeth [14].

Fluoride varnish application
Varnish is applied in the surgery. Application is simple and requires minimal training. OHEs and other dental care professionals (DCPs) can apply fluoride varnish to teeth when prescribed by a dentist if they have been trained to do so.

A thorough prophylaxis is not essential prior to application, but the removal of gross plaque is advised. Teeth should be dried with cotton rolls or a triple syringe, and a small quantity of varnish applied with a microbrush to pits, fissures, and interproximal surfaces (including carious lesions). The patient should avoid eating, drinking, and toothbrushing for 30 minutes after application and only eat soft foods for several hours after. Brushing can recommence on the following day.

The OHE should also be aware that certain varnishes contain alcohol, but the West Midlands Shari'ah Council has deemed them suitable for use by Muslims if used in small amounts [14].

Tablets or drops
Between the 1970s and 1990s, fluoride tablets and drops were widely recommended by the UK dental profession as an acceptable means of providing systemic fluoride for children with the additional topical benefits. However, the administration of these supplements is no longer considered to be an effective public health measure.

Since the introduction and widespread use of fluoride toothpaste, many experts believe that these supplements (containing sodium fluoride in 0.5 and 1 mg concentrations) should only be recommended when there is a medical history indicating that dental treatment is to be avoided wherever possible (e.g. cardiac, haemophiliac, severely physically/mentally disabled patients, or patients with a family history of caries).

Fluoridated milk
Fluoridated milk in UK schools was once advocated as an alternative means of giving fluoride by the *Borrow Milk Foundation* (a registered UK charity). The problem with this mode of administration is the variable uptake, since not all children drink milk and it is also only consumed during term-time.

There are still schemes in the UK, which supply school children with fluoridated milk in regions which are not fluoridated and where caries levels are high. However, children should not take part if they use fluoride tablets/rinses on a daily basis [10].

Fluoridated salt

This method is used in Switzerland, Hungary, France, and Germany. The promotion of salt has wider health implications and may result in conflict with other health messages.

Points to consider when recommending supplements

If fluoride supplements are recommended, the following points should be taken into account:

- Safe amounts of fluoride supplements can only be recommended if the level of fluoride in the water supply is known.
- Maximum benefit likely only if administered between 6 months and 13 years old.
- Critical level for fluorosis is between the ages of 15–30 months.
- Must not be administered at the same time of day as fluoride toothpaste.
- If one dose is missed, it must not be doubled the next day.
- Do not use if going on holiday – there may be fluoride in destination's water.

Table 11.1 shows the recommended daily doses for fluoride supplements.

Patients recommended for fluoride supplements

Patients who are particularly recommended to receive fluoride supplements include:

- Children at risk in areas with suboptimal water fluoride levels.
- Medically/physically compromised children (e.g. children that are not likely to be cooperative towards dental treatment and haemophiliacs).
- Children with siblings who have a high caries rate.

Dental fluorosis

Dental fluorosis (Figure 11.2 a,b) occurs when too much systemic fluoride is ingested, and presents dentally as opaque or white areas and lines or flecks on the enamel surface. It is most noticeable in the anterior regions.

Table 11.1 Recommended daily doses for fluoride supplements.

Age	Fluoride level below 0.3 ppm	Fluoride level between 0.3–0.7 ppm	Fluoride level over 0.7 ppm
6 months to 3 years	0.25 mg	None	None
3–6 years	0.5 mg	0.25 mg	None
Over 6 years	1 mg	0.5 mg	None

FLUORIDE

(a)

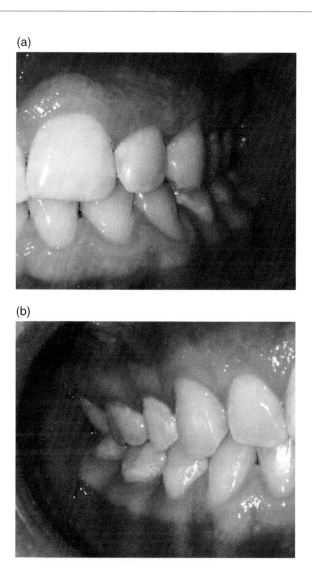

(b)

Figure 11.2 (a,b) Mild fluorosis. Source: Alison Chapman.

In geographical areas where water has high naturally occurring fluoride (in excess of 7 ppm), as seen in parts of India for example, it can result in very unsightly, yellow/brown pitted teeth. In the UK, these opaque or white areas on teeth are not always the result of ingesting too much fluoride but can be due to a number of causes (e.g. enamel faults caused by high temperatures and fever during tooth development). Table 11.2 highlights the association between levels of fluoride in water and fluorosis.

If a child ingests fluoride in excess, usually by swallowing toothpaste in larger quantities than the recommended pea-sized quantity from a brush, fluorosis can occur. This risk increases in areas where the water is fluoridated or

Table 11.2 The association between levels of fluoride in water and fluorosis.

Level of fluorosis	PPM in water	Effect on tooth
None	<1 ppm	None.
Not significant	1 ppm	No significant mottling and around 50% caries reduction.
Very mild	2 ppm	Small white opaque patches.
Mild	2–3 ppm	White opaque area involving half the crown.
Moderate	3–4 ppm	White opacity of crown and some brown mottling.
Severe	>4 ppm	White opacity of whole crown, brown mottling and pitting and hypoplasia.

when a child is receiving fluoride supplements. The greatest risk of fluorosis is between 15 and 30 months of age, when teeth are developing.

Fluoride swallowed in excessive quantities can be extremely toxic, particularly to small children, and if an overdose is suspected, the immediate antidote is for the child to drink milk and be taken to hospital as quickly as possible.

REFERENCES

1. Collins, W.J., Walsh, T. & Figures, K. (1999) *A Handbook for Dental Hygienists*, 4th edn. Butterworth Heinemann, Oxford.
2. Fejerskov, O. & Kidd, E. (2004) *Dental Caries: The Disease and Its Clinical Management*. Blackwell Munksgaard, Oxford.
3. The British Fluoridation Society (1983) *Comments on the Case Mrs Catherine McColl v Strathclyde Regional Council Held in the Court of Session, Edinburgh*. Liverpool: Department of Clinical Dental Sciences, University of Liverpool.
4. British Fluoridation Society (1985) *A Summary of the Knox Report and How It Refutes the Alleged Fluoridation – Cancer Link*. Liverpool: Department of Clinical Dental Sciences, University of Liverpool.
5. British Fluoridation Society (2005) *Water Fluoridation: A Briefing on the York University Systematic Review and Subsequent Research Developments*. Liverpool: Department of Clinical Dental Sciences, University of Liverpool.
6. In their element series three, Fluorine: Chemistry's Tiger. BBC Radio 4 [radio broadcast]. 3 April 2019. Available at: www.bbc.co.uk/programmes/b0bbrc0r [accessed 3 April 2019].
7. World Health Organization (2006) *Global consultation on oral health through fluoride, 2006*. Available at: www.who.int/oral_health/events/Global_consultation/en/ [accessed 2 May 2019].
8. World Health Organization (1994) *Fluorides and oral health. Technical Report Series No. 846*. Geneva: WHO.
9. Petersen, P.E. & Lennon, M.A. (2004) *Effective use of fluorides for the prevention of dental caries in the 21st century: the WHO approach*. Community Dentistry and Oral Epidemiology, 32, 319–321.

FLUORIDE

10. Public Health England. (2018) *Water fluoridation: health monitoring report for England 2018*. Available at: www.gov.uk/government/publications/water-fluoridation-health-monitoring-report-for-england-2018 [accessed 30 April 2019].

11. Cochrane (2015) *Water fluoridation to prevent tooth decay*. Available at: www.cochrane.org/CD010856/ORAL_water-fluoridation-prevent-tooth-decay [accessed 10 June 2019].

12. Drinking Water Inspectorate (2016) *Code of Practice on Technical Aspects of Fluoridation of Water Supplies 2016*. Available at: http://dwi.defra.gov.uk/stakeholders/information-letters/2016/01-2016-annexa.pdf [accessed 30 April 2019].

13. Drinking Water Inspectorate (2020) *Typical fluoride levels in zones during 2012*. Available at: www.dwi.gov.uk/consumers/advice-leaflets/fluoridemap.pdf [accessed 24 January 2020].

14. Public Health England and Department of Health (2017) *Delivering better oral health: an evidence-based toolkit for prevention*. Available at: www.gov.uk/government/publications/delivering-better-oral-health-an-evidence-based-toolkit-for-prevention [accessed 30 April 2019].

FLUORIDE

Chapter 12

Fissure sealants

Learning outcomes

By the end of this chapter you should be able to:

1. Define what a *fissure sealant* is and explain why it is used.
2. Identify sites most commonly sealed and materials/systems used.
3. Describe the fissure sealing technique.
4. List trials on the effectiveness of fissure sealants.

WHAT IS A FISSURE SEALANT?

A fissure sealant is a plastic resin material that is placed in the pits, fissures, and buccal grooves of molar teeth (less common in premolars), and the cingulums and palatal grooves of incisors, in order to prevent or arrest the development of caries.

Fissure sealants were first developed in the 1970s as a preventive measure. Unlike amalgam restorations, there is no preparatory cutting or drilling of the enamel surface of the tooth unless caries is present.

Reasons for using fissure sealants

Fissure sealants make teeth easier to clean and protect surfaces from plaque. Fissures in newly erupted permanent molars are often too small to be penetrated by toothbrush bristles and plaque can get trapped in them, which can lead to the development of caries.

The Child Dental Health Survey 2013 survey found that approximately 31% of 5 year olds and 46% of 8 year olds had obvious decay in their primary teeth [1]. A recent Cochrane report (on 15 studies comparing the effectiveness of resin-based sealants to no sealants) found that: *'children who had sealant*

Basic Guide to Oral Health Education and Promotion, Third Edition.
Alison Chapman and Simon H. Felton.
© 2021 John Wiley & Sons Ltd. Published 2021 by John Wiley & Sons Ltd.
Companion website: www.wiley.com/go/felton/oralhealth

applied to their back teeth were less likely to have tooth decay in their back teeth than children with no sealant' [2].

When and where to seal

Fissure sealing can be carried out in older children and adults, and is most effective when placed during the early months after eruption (i.e. when the enamel is not fully mature). Enamel is not fully hardened by the time of tooth eruption. Maturation (hardening) of the enamel takes several years to complete, and the probability of a caries attack reaches a peak at 2–4 years post-eruption. Fissure sealants are sometimes carried out in teenage children, as soon as the second molars (*sevens*) erupt.

Fissure sealants are most commonly used in the following cases:

- Fully erupted teeth (usually 6s and 7s) with no flaps or contamination from saliva, which could result in failure of the sealant.
- Sticky fissures susceptible to food debris and bacteria in children.
- Deep cingulums, and buccal or palatal grooves.
- Patients where a high caries risk is indicated/history of caries in deciduous teeth.
- High caries incidence in siblings.
- Patients with a serious medical condition (e.g. congenital heart disease, haemophilia) who need to avoid dental extractions.
- Patients who are unable to cope with adequate cleaning and dental treatment.

Fissure sealant materials/systems

Sealants are divided into two groups: filled and unfilled. Some sealants, which are filled with lithium alumina silicate, are more resistant to abrasion, have a prolonged life, and are easier to see in the tooth [3].

There are several materials in common use. The glass-ionomer cement (GIC) is sometimes used, but has been shown to be less effective than composite resins (largely because appointment-keeping is poor) [4]. However, glass ionomers are effective as temporary sealants in uncooperative patients or those with partially erupted teeth, and can be placed in the presence of saliva. Tooth-coloured sealants are considered to be better cosmetically, but clear sealants allow for inspection, which is particularly useful if previously undiagnosed caries is present.

The more commonly used composite resins can be used in several ways:

- Two solutions are mixed together and polymerized by chemical reaction (rarely used).
- Light-polymerized sealants. These are applied and sealed by a quartz halogen bulb, which is considered safer than plasma lights and ultraviolet lights (now considered obsolete).

Self-etching systems are under trial but appear to give inferior retention. They should be restricted to uncooperative patients and regarded as temporary.

Preventive resin restorations (PRRs) should be used where pits and fissures are decayed. The carious area should be cleaned and filled with a glass ionomer and then the non-carious area should be fissure-sealed.

It is essential to check fissure sealants regularly, and any defects in the sealant should be repaired to prevent leakage and bacterial invasion.

Sealant placement

Oral health educators (OHEs) may need to explain the sealant procedure to parents, and must therefore be familiar with the technique, although it is not the role of the OHE to carry out treatment.

The professional undertaking the procedure should read the instructions on the box, which are generally as follows:

1. Identify the tooth/teeth to be sealed (Figure 12.1a).
2. Clean the area to remove plaque. As residues may be left, it is probably better not to use pastes or pumice.
3. Isolate the tooth with a rubber dam (often not tolerated well by small children), or cotton wool rolls. Dry the tooth surface with oil-free air.
4. Etch the surface of the tooth for 15–20 seconds with phosphoric acid (35% solution) (Figure 12.1b).
5. Wash the surface with an air syringe for 15 seconds, taking care to avoid contamination from saliva, which is the most common reason for the failure of fissure sealants.
6. Replace the isolation of the tooth using fresh, dry cotton wool rolls and a saliva ejector. Dry the tooth (Figure 12.1c), and ensure the surface has a frosted appearance. If not, then re-etch the tooth using 35% phosphoric acid concentration for 10 seconds, then repeat rinsing and replace the isolation.
7. Apply sealant, taking care that it flows across the surface in one direction (to avoid air bubbles). Remove any air bubbles carefully with a probe.
8. Polymerize using a white light for 20–30 seconds.
9. Check the integrity of the sealant and the bite – no need to adjust, as the sealant wears down fairly quickly (Figure 12.1d).
10. Check interdentally with floss.

Tips on fissure sealing in children

Fissure sealants are the first clinical intervention in the dental chair for many children, while some children may have already had a troublesome prior experience of dentistry, such as extraction under general anaesthesia. The OHE may therefore be able to help with calming small children.

FISSURE SEALANTS

(a)

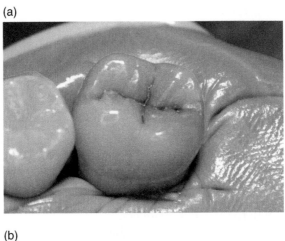

(b)

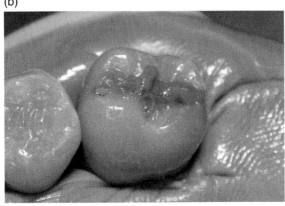

Figure 12.1 Teeth to be (a) sealed, (b) etched, (c) dried and (d) sealed. Source: Alison Chapman.

The OHE can explain that:

- They will need to sit still for a couple of minutes for each tooth, with an opportunity to 'have a wriggle' between sealing teeth.
- A big, wide mouth will help the operator see the teeth at the back.

If time permits, show children the equipment that will be used:

- The air/water syringe and sealing light.
- Demonstrate suction on their hand, explaining that it is like a noisy vacuum cleaner.
- Show them the acid etch, *'it tastes like sour sweets'*, so keep the tongue away!
- Cotton wool rolls used to keep the tongue away – explain the sensation (dry, firm, etc.).

(c)

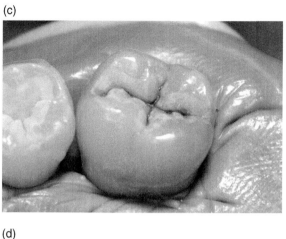

(d)

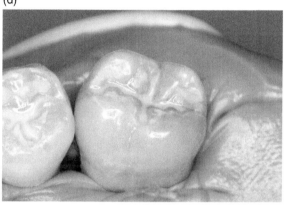

Figure 12.1 (Continued)

Further advice

All patients should be given further preventive advice at the same time as sealants are applied, including:

- Diet – e.g. frequency of sugar, with an aim to reduce total sugar intake (see Chapter 9).
- Effective oral hygiene regimen (e.g. size of toothbrush head, frequency of toothbrushing).
- Use of fluoride and suitable toothpastes (1000 ppm for under 3 year olds, 1500 ppm for over 3 year olds). Enamel maturation is more rapid in the presence of fluoride, so all children should use fluoride toothpaste to assist this process as well to help prevent caries. Fluoride applied topically helps strengthen enamel and interferes with bacterial reproduction (see Chapter 11).

- Consider prescribing high fluoride toothpaste: 2800 ppm for patients 10 years and over, and 5000 ppm for patients 16 and over.

Clinical trials

Clinical trials (and reviews), which can be used as evidence of the effectiveness of fissure sealing in preventing the development of caries, have been carried out by:

- British Society for Paediatric Dentistry (BSPD) [5].
- Rock et al. [6].
- British Association for the Study of Community Dentistry [7].
- Cochrane review [2].

REFERENCES

1. NHS Digital (2015) *Child Dental Health Survey 2013, England, Wales and Northern Ireland.* Available at: https://digital.nhs.uk/data-and-information/publications/statistical/children-s-dental-health-survey/child-dental-health-survey-2013-england-wales-and-northern-ireland [accessed 18 March 2019].
2. Cochrane (2017) *Sealants for preventing tooth decay in permanent teeth.* Available at: www.cochrane.org/CD001830/ORAL_sealants-preventing-tooth-decay-permanent-teeth [accessed January 15 2020].
3. Collins, W.J., Walsh, T., & Figures, K. (1999). *A Handbook for Dental Hygienists*, 4th edn. Butterworth Heinemann, Oxford.
4. Chadwick, B. (2005) A randomised controlled trial to determine the effectiveness of glass ionomer sealants in pre-school children. *Caries Research* 39, 34–40.
5. British Association for Study of Paediatric Dentistry. (2006) A randomised controlled trial of the effectiveness of a one-step conditioning agent in sealant placement: 6 month results. *International Journal of Paediatric Dentistry* 16, 424–430.
6. Rock, W.P. & Evans, R.I.W. (1983) A comparative study between chemically polymerized fissure sealant and a light-cured resin. *British Dental Journal* 155, 344–346.
7. Pitts, N.B., Evans, D.J. & Nugen, Z.J. (1996) The dental caries experience of 14-year-old children in the United Kingdom. Surveys coordinated by the British Association for the Study of Community Dentistry in 1994/1995. *Community Dental Health* 13, 51–58.

FISSURE SEALANTS

Chapter 13

Smoking cessation and substance misuse

Learning outcomes

By the end of this chapter you should be able to:

1. List reasons why people use tobacco and its effects on general and oral health.
2. List common types of nicotine replacement therapy (NRT) available.
3. Provide advice, support, and signposting on changing habits and smoking cessation.
4. Detail other drug misuse and their effects on oral health.
5. Provide guidance on recommended alcohol limits, plus advice, support and signposting on alcohol and illegal drug misuse.

SMOKING AND TOBACCO USE

Tobacco use is a significant public health problem worldwide and is a leading cause of preventable death and disease. According to the World Health Organization (WHO), tobacco kills over 7 million people each year [1].

Smoking rates vary across the UK population, and are highest in the lowest income groups. In England, for example, rates of smoking have declined steadily from 28% (1998) to 18% (2015); 19% of men and 17% of women being current smokers, and 5% of adults use e-cigarettes, otherwise known as vaping [2]. However, despite this decline, tobacco use continues to be a factor in the deaths of over 70 000 people every year (1900 of these from mouth cancer) [3].

The use of smokeless tobacco and/or betel nut chewing (betel leaf mixed with areca nut, also known as *paan*), is common amongst certain ethnic minority groups and can have similar effects to tobacco smoking (see Chapter 25).

Basic Guide to Oral Health Education and Promotion, Third Edition.
Alison Chapman and Simon H. Felton.
© 2021 John Wiley & Sons Ltd. Published 2021 by John Wiley & Sons Ltd.
Companion website: www.wiley.com/go/felton/oralhealth

The Oral Health Educator (OHE), like other dental care professionals (DCPs) and health workers, is in a prime position to help receptive patients stop using tobacco (cigarettes, shisha, cigars, chewing tobacco, or paan), by providing brief interventions and signposting them towards stop smoking services and, in doing so, improve both their oral and general health.

Effects of tobacco on oral health

Tobacco use increases the risk of the following oral diseases and conditions:

- Mouth cancer (see Chapter 8).
- Destruction of the periodontium (see Chapter 4).
- Delayed healing following extractions.
- *Dry socket* following extractions.
- Tooth loss.
- Stickier plaque – leading to gingivitis/periodontitis (see Chapters 3 and 4).
- Stained teeth (see Chapter 2).
- Halitosis.
- Xerostomia (see Chapter 7).
- Black hairy tongue (see Chapter 8).
- Loss of taste (and smell).

Effects of tobacco on general health

The OHE also needs to know the potential effects of tobacco on general health, in order to help change patients' attitudes.

Conditions and consequences include:

- Chronic bronchitis, emphysema, and chronic obstructive pulmonary disorder (COPD).
- Cardiovascular disease (CVD) – the biggest single killer in the UK, including coronary heart disease (angina and heart attacks) and strokes.
- Infertility.
- Certain cancers – particularly of the lung, mouth, larynx, oesophagus, and bladder. The combined effects of smoking and moderate/high alcohol consumption (particularly spirits) increase the likelihood of cancer (see Chapter 8).
- Miscarriage, premature birth, ectopic pregnancy, small head circumference, and low birth weight.
- Passive smoking is especially dangerous in children and can increase the risk of:
  - Childhood cancers and leukaemia.
  - Sudden infant death syndrome (*cot death*).

- Middle ear infection (*glue ear*).
- Poor lung function.
- Respiratory conditions – e.g. asthma, bronchitis, and pneumonia.

Reasons why people use tobacco

Many people who use tobacco want to stop. They have the knowledge about why they should give up, but not the willpower to do so and require a change in attitude.

Attitudes are formed from personal experiences throughout life and encompass influences from family and friends, values and beliefs. Patients must have a strong desire to change their behaviour before they will do so. In order to influence them to quit, the OHE needs to have some knowledge of the main reasons why people use tobacco:

- They are addicted. Many people in this group want to change their behaviour, yet cannot break the habit
- It makes them feel grown up amongst their peers (pre-teens/younger teenagers).
- To relieve stress (even though nicotine is actually a stimulant). This is the most common reason the OHE will be given, and the usual reason for a relapse.
- To keep weight down.
- Social reasons. They may have the odd cigarette on an evening out, but are not addicted.

Helping patients change their habits

OHEs are in a prime position to offer help to patients wishing to change their tobacco habit and, like other DCPs and health professionals, have a duty of care to do so, as well as checking their smoking status annually.

However, more detailed advice and support should only be provided by dental staff that have completed a recognised cessation training programme, such as that run by the National Centre for Smoking Cessation and Training (NCSCT), which offers online learning suitable for all DCPs in England, Wales, Ireland, and for the Armed Forces in the rest of the world. It is also worth contacting your local stop smoking service, which may also provide training and further information that can be given to patients [4].

Patients will only change their behaviour if they have the knowledge to do so, and their attitude is geared towards a behavioural change.

Guidelines for brief intervention

In most cases, the OHE will be delivering very brief advice (VBA) to tobacco users, and it is recommended that they use the following pathway developed by the NCSCT to maximise the chance of a successful quit attempt, which can be delivered in less than 30 seconds [4]:

1. Establish and record smoking status (**Ask**):
   * All patients should be asked about their tobacco use (past and present) annually by a member of the dental team and their notes updated.
   * Simply ask, '*Do you want to stop smoking/chewing tobacco?*'
2. Advising on the personal benefits of quitting (**Advise**):
   * If they want to quit, advise them that the best way to stop is with a combination of support and treatment.
   Do not:
   * Warn them of the dangers and advise to stop – as this can create a defensive reaction/anxiety and be time-consuming (leave this to the stop smoking service).
   * Ask how long they have used tobacco/which type/how much they use.
3. Offering help (**Act**).
   * All users should receive advice about the value of attending their local stop smoking services for specialised help. Those who are interested and motivated to stop should be referred to these services.
   * For patients who do not want to stop, say something like: '*that's ok, but help will always be available, just let me know if you change your mind*'.

Harm reduction

Harm reduction involves using licensed nicotine-containing and/or pharmaco-therapy (prescription only) product(s) to reduce tobacco use.

Most health problems associated with smoking (and tobacco use) are caused by other components in tobacco, not by the (addictive) nicotine component. It is therefore safer to use a licensed nicotine-containing and/or a craving-reduction product than to smoke. NRT products have been demonstrated in trials to be safe to use for at least 5 years [5].

In fact, people who just reduce the amount they use without supplementing their nicotine intake with a licensed nicotine product tend to compensate by inhaling smoke deeper into their lungs and taking more puffs. And so, it is recommended that they reduce the number of cigarettes and use a licensed therapeutic product, thus changing their behaviour. Patients should be advised that by reducing their usage with NRT that they are more likely to stop in the future [6].

Recommended harm reduction products

Types of products recommended, and currently available, at NHS stop smoking services include [7]:

SMOKING CESSATION AND
SUBSTANCE MISUSE

- NRT (unprescribed/prescribed products containing nicotine):
  - Gum.
  - Patches.
  - Lozenges.
  - Nasal spray.
  - Inhalator (*plastic* cigarette).
  - Microtabs (dissolve under the tongue).
- Pharmacotherapy products:
  - Varenicline (Champix®) tablets.
  - Bupropion (Zyban™) tablets.

While NRT products are widely available over-the-counter, it is still recommended that patients are advised to discuss the most appropriate product and usage with a healthcare professional (like their GP, or at a stop smoking service).

Pharmacotherapy products must be prescribed by a doctor, due to their potential side effects and interaction with other medications. For example, Zyban is not available for pregnant patients, or those with a history of depression or taking antidepressants.

Remember! The OHE should signpost patients/ask for help from professionals with more experience if they feel out of their depth when advising patients who want to stop smoking.

Advice on vaping (e-cigarettes)

The use of, and experimentation with, e-cigarettes is increasingly common, and government stances on use vary. For example, some countries have amended their policies to restrict their use, while others, such as Canada and New Zealand, promote their use as a harm reduction method [8]. In the US, a 2018 study has found that the viscosity of e-liquids and some classes of chemicals in sweet flavours may increase the risk of caries [8].

At the time of writing there are no medicinally licensed e-cigarettes in the UK, or the rest of the world. In the UK, the government is committed to more research into whether their use can be included in harm reduction, but smokers who use vaping should be advised to quit smoking. Data from stop smoking services in England, suggests that using e-cigarettes as part of a quitting smoking attempt remains the main reason for vaping and is helpful for attendees [9].

The government therefore advises that combining vaping (the most popular source of support used by smokers in the general population), with stop smoking service support (the most effective type of support), should be a recommended option available to all smokers and stop smoking practitioners, and health professionals should provide behavioural support to smokers who want to use an e-cigarette to help them quit smoking. Again, online training is available from the NCSCT.

Pregnant patients should be advised not to use e-cigarettes that contain nicotine because it is highly addictive and can be harmful to the unborn child.

Summary of advice

Summary of advice for patients who smoke and who are using, or are interested in using an e-cigarette to quit smoking [5]:

- Products are not licensed medicines, but regulated by the Tobacco and Related Products Regulations 2016.
- Many people have found them helpful to quit smoking.
- Evidence suggests that e-cigarettes are less harmful than smoking, but not risk-free [4].
- Evidence on any effects of e-cigarettes on long-term health is still developing.
- Should stop using tobacco at the same time.

The process of change

The chances of smoking cessation for many patients increase significantly when nicotine addiction is managed alongside a change in behaviour to their general lifestyle. It can be useful for patients to make a list of why they want to stop, positives it will bring, and change other habits, such as getting more exercise, drinking less alcohol, and improving diet, although too much change at once can be detrimental.

By studying the theory of changing behaviour, the OHE will have a better knowledge on the stages people go through when quitting.

The OHE should therefore follow the pathway as outlined in the *Smokefree and Smiling* NHS publication [3], as well as familiarising themselves with Prochaska and DiClemente's Process of Change (see following text).

Prochaska and DiClemente's Process of Change

In 1986, two educators called Prochaska and DiClemente developed a theory called the *Process of Change* [10]. They believed that changing attitudes and behaviour is a continuous cycle, rather than a single occurrence. Their theories can be applied to many circumstances, smoking cessation being just one example. Many patients regard stopping their habit as a one-off event and see the resumption of the habit as failure. The OHE's role is to help patients see it as a continual process (Figure 13.1).

The stages of the cycle, and an example of each stage (related in this case to smoking) are shown in italics.

1. Thinking about change:

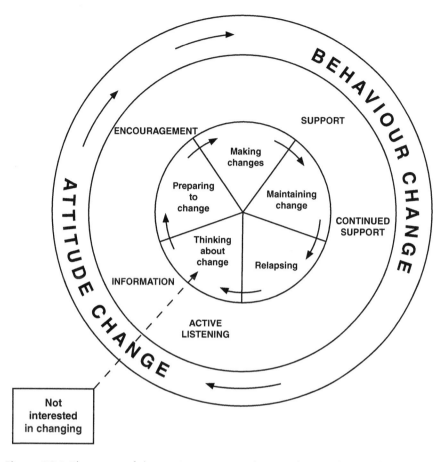

Figure 13.1 The process of change. Source: From Ruth McIntosh. Reproduced with permission of Ruth McIntosh.

   Concerned smoker – worried about the effects of smoking or thinking of quitting.

2. Preparing to change:
   Planning to quit – getting ready to quit – setting a quit date.

3. Making the change:
   Action (quit day) – actually stopping smoking.

4. Maintaining the change:
   Maintain a quit attempt – resisting relapse.

5. Relapse:
   Has gone back to smoking – could be temporary or long term.

   The important thing for the OHE to stress is that a relapse is not the end of the cycle, but the part that precedes beginning again. Be prepared to spend time listening, talking and empathising with patients, but never be judgemental or patronising; some smokers are contented and not interested in quitting. The OHE will encounter resentment if they apply pressure for change.

Patients who decide to stop will need:

- Empathy (includes active listening).
- Understanding (includes giving accurate information or signposting appropriately).
- Encouragement (it helps to know that your dentist and staff really care).
- Support (often over a long period). Patients need to know that they can come back to the OHE when their resolve weakens, or life events increase their stress.

OTHER DRUG MISUSE AND SUPPORT

Oral health problems are also very common amongst patients who misuse/abuse alcohol and other drugs. Not only can the effect of the drug itself cause oral health conditions, but the fact that users often have a poor oral health regime.

The OHE should therefore be aware of the effects of alcohol and other drugs on the oral cavity, provide basic oral health advice to improve hygiene, and be able to signpost users to their GP and other specialist services to get help with their addiction.

Alcohol

Alcohol abuse is a widespread problem, and its effects on the body and society are wide ranging and well documented.

Together with smoking, alcohol is a main cause of mouth cancer [4] (see Chapter 8), as well as being a factor in tooth surface loss through erosion (see Chapter 6). When both alcohol and tobacco are used together, the risks on the oral health are multiplied, accounting for the majority of mouth cancer cases. Further, it is estimated that heavy drinkers and smokers have a much greater risk of developing mouth cancer than those who neither smoke nor drink more than two units of alcohol a day. Excessive alcohol intake is also associated with dental trauma through injury.

What is a unit of alcohol?
One unit of alcohol is 10 mL of pure alcohol.

The unit(s) of alcohol in a drink can be worked out by multiplying the percentage of alcohol by the quantity and dividing by 1000. For example, a pint of strong beer could be: 5 (%) × 568 (mL) ÷ 1000 = 2.84 units

One unit is roughly equal to:

- Half a pint of beer/lager/cider (3–4%).
- 25 mL glass of spirits.
- 50 mL of port or sherry.

For wine:

- 175 mL glass of ordinary strength = 2.3 units.
- 250 mL (large glass) of ordinary strength = 3.3 units.

Recommended limit

The OHE should be able to advise patients on the recommended alcohol limits, which in the UK are currently not to regularly drink more than 14 units per week, which is the equivalent of either:

- Six pints of (4%) beer.
- Six glasses of (175 mL, 13%) wine.
- Fourteen glasses of (25 mL, 40%) spirits.

Patients should be recommended that these units are best spread evenly across the week (limiting the amount drunk in each session), with several alcohol-free days each week.

Pregnant patients should be advised not to drink alcohol.

Guidelines for a brief intervention

As with tobacco use, the OHE is in a very good position to offer very brief advice (VBA) on drinking, and for all patients, they should [4]:

- **Ask** – Establish and record if the patient is drinking above recommended levels.
- **Advise** – offer very brief advice to those drinking above recommended levels.
- **Act** – refer or signpost high risk drinkers to their GP or local alcohol support services.

Further advice and support

Alcohol advice and support requires specialist care beyond the scope of the OHE, and the OHE should signpost willing patients who need help to their GP and/or the following bodies:

- Alcoholics Anonymous.
- Alcohol Change UK (a merger between Alcohol Concern and Alcohol Research UK).
- Drinkaware.

Illegal drug misuse

The OHE should be aware of the effects that illegal drugs can have on the oral cavity. Many users' oral health will suffer from the effects of a poor diet, frequent snacking, dry mouth, and high sugar consumption. Drug use can also mask dental pain in users, who may be unaware of a problem as a result.

The OHE can provide advice on improving oral health caused by these drugs, as they do in a general sense with other patients, but they must be aware that patients are unlikely to improve their oral hygiene and behaviour without first addressing the source of the problem (i.e. their addiction) with a specialist. It is therefore important to provide support and advice on oral care, and signpost known users who want to change their habit to their GP to receive specialist advice on treatment for their addiction.

Opiates (heroin, morphine) and methadone

The effects of opiates and methadone use on the oral cavity include:

- Tooth decay (see Chapter 5) – increased risk due to snacking (cravings).
- Bruxism, clenching, and grinding – leading to attrition and broken teeth.

Oral methadone is sometimes supplied as a sugary syrup to prevent intravenous abuse of the drug, but it should not be held in the mouth and the mouth should be rinsed afterwards with water. Patients should be encouraged to ask for sugar-free methadone, if they have been prescribed this drug.

Methadone is also acidic and can cause vomiting and reflux with associated oral health risks. Although it makes the user less hungry, it also causes them to crave sweets and carbonated drinks.

Cannabis

Many of the effects on the oral cavity are the same as with tobacco smoking and the OHE can provide advice and support based on the effects of tobacco. There is also an increased risk of tooth decay due to snacking (cravings).

Cocaine

The effects of cocaine use on the oral cavity include:

- Localised gum and bone damage due to rubbing cocaine onto the gums.
- Localised tooth decay due to street drugs being cut down with sugar/glucose powder.
- Spontaneous bleeding of the gums.
- Erosion and subsequent sensitivity of the buccal surfaces where the cocaine has been placed.
- Bruxism – clenching and grinding teeth, leading to attrition and broken teeth.
- When snorted it can damage the septum (the cartilage in the nose that separates the nostrils).

Cocaine can also interact with dental anaesthetics, and patients should be advised to refrain from taking cocaine before undergoing dental treatment.

Amphetamines and ecstasy

The effects of amphetamines and ecstasy on the oral cavity include:

- Xerostomia (see Chapter 7).
- Stimulate carbohydrate intake and thirst – again, particularly fizzy drinks, which can lead to erosion (see Chapter 6).
- Bruxism – clenching and grinding due to increased motor activity – can lead to attrition and broken teeth (see Chapter 6).

Hallucinogens (LSD, magic mushrooms, angel dust)

The effects of hallucinogens on the oral cavity include:

- Increased risk of mouth injuries from users who take more risks while under the influence.
- Bruxism – clenching and grinding leading to attrition and broken teeth.
- Panic attacks – induced by the dental setting.

Solvent abuse

The effects of solvent abuse on the oral cavity include:

- *Glue sniffer's rash* around the mouth and nose.
- *Oral frostbite* may be present from inhaling some aerosols. (The chemical propellant in the aerosol can cause burning of tissues similar to frost bite.)
- Inhalants can sensitise the heart muscle to adrenaline. Therefore, dental anaesthetics containing this should not be used on suspected solvent abusers.
- General anaesthetics should be avoided because of possible liver damage.

REFERENCES

1. World Health Organization (2019) *Tobacco.* Available at: www.who.int/newsroom/fact-sheets/detail/tobacco [accessed 10 May 2019].
2. NHS Digital (2016) *The Health Survey for England (2015).* Available at: https://webarchive.nationalarchives.gov.uk/20180307193646/http://digital.nhs.uk/catalogue/PUB22610 [accessed 4 April 2019].
3. Public Health England (2014) *Smokefree and smiling: Helping dental patients to quit tobacco.* Available at: www.gov.uk/government/publications/smokefree-and-smiling [accessed 15 May 2019].
4. Public Health England and Department of Health (2017) *Delivering better oral health: an evidence-based toolkit for prevention.* Available at: www.gov.uk/government/publications/delivering-better-oral-health-an-evidence-based-toolkit-for-prevention [accessed 30 April 2019].

5. NICE (2018) *Stop smoking interventions and services guideline [NG92]*. Available at: www.nice.org.uk/guidance/ng92/ [accessed May 14 2019].

6. NICE (2013) *Smoking: harm reduction Public health guideline [PH45]*. Available at: www.nice.org.uk/guidance/ph45 [accessed May 14 2019].

7. NHS (2019) Smokefree: *Stop smoking medicines*. Available at: www.nhs.uk/smokefree/help-and-advice/prescription-medicines. [accessed May 14 2019].

8. Kim, S.A., Smith, S., Beauchamp, C., Song, Y., Chiang, M., Giuseppetti, A. et al. (2018) Cariogenic potential of sweet flavors in electronic-cigarette liquids. *PLoS ONE* 13, e0203717. Available at: https://doi.org/10.1371/journal.pone.0203717 [accessed May 14 2019].

9. Public Health England (2019*) Vaping in England: evidence update summary February 2019*. Available at: www.gov.uk/government/publications/vaping-in-england-an-evidence-update-february-2019/ [accessed 15 May 2019].

10. Ireland, R. (2004) *Advanced Dental Nursing*. Blackwell Science Ltd, Oxford.

SMOKING CESSATION AND
SUBSTANCE MISUSE

Chapter 14

Anti-plaque agents

Learning outcomes

By the end of this chapter you should be able to:

1. List anti-plaque agents and discuss different types with patients.
2. State the types, constituents and functions of toothpaste.
3. State the types, recommended usage, and side effects of mouthwashes.
4. List the functions and benefits of sugar-free chewing gum.

INTRODUCTION

Anti-plaque agents (particularly, toothpastes, mouthwashes, and chewing gum) have been a large growth industry in the UK consumer market.

In view of the role of bacterial plaque in periodontal disease, clinicians and manufacturers have been interested in the potential value of anti-plaque/anti-bacterial agents in both toothpastes and mouthwashes, and there are now so many on the market that patients (and dental professionals!) can become confused. They will often ask oral health educators (OHEs) what toothpastes and mouthwashes they recommend, and it is therefore important to know some background information about the most frequently used products.

Toothpaste

Toothpaste comes in the form of pastes, gels, or striped combinations of the two, and manufacturers compete with each other to include new ingredients in their products. There are now different anti-plaque and anti-calculus agents; fluoride in most pastes; a range of products for sensitivity and dry mouths; whitening and anti-erosion properties, and homeopathic pastes for those seeking no chemical additives.

Basic Guide to Oral Health Education and Promotion, Third Edition.
Alison Chapman and Simon H. Felton.
© 2021 John Wiley & Sons Ltd. Published 2021 by John Wiley & Sons Ltd.
Companion website: www.wiley.com/go/felton/oralhealth

It is impossible to advise the OHE on what to recommend to patients, and the dental professional will often be guided by what the dentist suggests and what the practice sells. If patients have always used a particular brand, they will probably not want to be persuaded otherwise. However, OHEs should stress the benefits of fluoride in toothpaste, particularly for children (see Chapter 11).

Children up to the age of 3 years old should use a smear of toothpaste containing 1000 ppm and adults should ensure that the paste is not swallowed in large amounts. Children over 3 years old and adults should use a pea-sized amount of toothpaste containing 1350–1500 ppm [1].

Toothpastes with a greater concentration of fluoride, 2800 ppm (for high caries risk patients aged 10 years or over), and 5000 ppm (for high caries risk patients over 16 years), are available on NHS prescription.

Constituents of toothpaste

Toothpaste contains as many as 20 different ingredients, but the main ones are:

- Polishing agents – mild abrasives to remove/reduce plaque debris and stains (e.g. calcium carbonate, dehydrated silica gels, hydrated aluminium oxides, magnesium carbonate, phosphate salts, and silicates).
- Binding agent – controls stability, consistency, and dispersion of paste in the mouth (e.g. seaweed extracts, cellulose, silica).
- Foaming agent – a mild detergent that lowers surface tension and loosens debris, aids dispersion, and has psychological benefits (mouth feels clean). It is usually sodium lauryl sulphate (this reacts with chlorhexidine, which is why patients are advised not to use toothpaste and mouthwash at the same time). Some patients may find that they develop ulcers if this is included in their toothpaste (see Chapter 8).
- Humectant – reduces moisture loss, sweetens, and keeps consistency (e.g. glycerine, sorbitol).
- Flavouring (often peppermint or spearmint) – masks the flavour of other components and important to consumer. It can be difficult to find non-mint flavours, in which case recommend homeopathic toothpastes, which can be found in health shops.
- Therapeutic agents:
  - Fluoride – Sodium fluoride, sodium monofluorophosphate, stannous fluoride. Quantities in non-prescription toothpastes are regulated to 1500 ppm maximum for adults and 1000 ppm for children under 3 years old.
  - Desensitising agents – such as strontium chloride, strontium acetate, potassium nitrate, potassium citrate, arginine, and calcium carbonate (e.g. Colgate® Pro-Relief™).
  - Anti-plaque agents – e.g. triclosan.
  - Anti-calculus agents – e.g. pyrophosphates, ureates, zinc citrate.
  - Bicarbonates – reduce the acidity of plaque.

ANTI-PLAQUE AGENTS

Functions of toothpaste

There are six principal functions of toothpaste (in conjunction with toothbrushing):

1. Minimises plaque and calculus build-up (plaque-removing agents). Some pastes contain chlorhexidine, which is effective but can stain. Sodium bicarbonate (baking soda) is gentler, but less effective and many patients do not like the taste.
2. Increasing resistance of the tooth to decay (fluoride). Different forms of fluoride are present in different pastes, the most common being sodium monofluoro-phosphate. Some pastes contain sodium fluoride or stannous fluoride.
3. Removing food debris. Many patients like the foaming action of tooth-paste caused by mild detergents (usually sodium lauryl sulfate). It is important to stress that an effective method of brushing is equally impor-tant in removing food particles.
4. Freshening the mouth. Various agents are added to flavour and sweeten pastes (sugar was once used!). Now sweeteners are used – usually soluble saccharin or xylitol (see Chapter 10) – and flavourings as mentioned previously.
5. Desensitising (strontium chloride/potassium chloride). Around two-thirds of adults in the UK have wear into dentine on their anterior teeth, which can cause tooth sensitivity (see Chapter 6).
6. Whitening. Patients invariably want whiter teeth and may ask the OHE's advice. It should be explained that whatever the toothpaste manufacturer's claims, these toothpastes do not change the colour of teeth, but assist in removing extrinsic protein stains. If a patient is very concerned about the colour of their teeth, suggest a consultation with the dentist (see Chapter 2).

Advising on toothpastes

When advising on toothpastes at the request of a patient:

- Promote a good quality paste with fluoride.
- Be aware of different ingredients in pastes, which claim to reduce plaque (patients often ask for advice on this).
- Be prepared to recommend pastes to help sensitivity (patients often ask how they work and this should be explained in simple terms).
- Be aware of homeopathic toothpastes.

Homeopathic toothpastes

Some patients will ask about homeopathic toothpastes, which can be obtained from health food shops. It is now possible to obtain homeopathic toothpaste with added fluoride, but the patient should be warned that they do not always contain fluoride. If not, the patient should use a daily fluoride mouthwash to combat the loss (see also Chapter 19).

These pastes are often manufactured without mint or other strong flavours, which many patients find more acceptable. Aloe vera (an ingredient) has anti-bacterial qualities, and can help with ailments such as angular cheilitis (see Chapter 8).

Anti-plaque mouthwashes

An anti-plaque mouthwash is an agent that is capable of reducing gingivitis. If the product claims to reduce plaque, that does not necessarily mean that it will be sufficient to reduce gum disease. It is important to look for proportional differences in claims.

Besides the treatment of gingivitis, mouthwashes can also be used as an adjunct for the treatment of periodontitis, pericoronitis (infection around wisdom teeth), dental caries, sensitivity, and other more serious conditions of the oral mucosa. Chlorhexidine gluconate is considered the gold standard by which all other mouthwashes are measured (see following text).

Chlorhexidine gluconate

Chlorhexidine gluconate has a broad anti-microbial spectrum and is active on both gram-positive and gram-negative bacteria.

It has been shown in long-term studies to reduce plaque and gingivitis by an average of 55% and 45% respectively [2]. Thirty per cent of a chlorhexidine gluconate mouthwash is retained in the mouth, and elevated levels are found in saliva after 24 hours.

Forms of chlorhexidine gluconate

Forms of chlorhexidine gluconate include:

- Mouthwash (0.2% chlorhexidine gluconate) – rinse for 1 minute every 12 hours. Several mouthwashes on the market contain chlorhexidine gluconate, and there is an alcohol-free chlorhexidine mouthwash following public concern that alcohol in mouthwashes could cause cancer.
- Gel (1% chlorhexidine gluconate) – applied topically.
- Spray (0.2% chlorhexidine gluconate).
- Chewing gum.
- Toothpaste.
- Slow release chip (e.g. PerioChip®) – placed in deep pockets by the dentist or hygienist.

When advising patients about the use of chlorhexidine gluconate mouthwash, after brushing they should rinse thoroughly with water and leave at least a 5-minute gap before rinsing with chlorhexidine. This is because the reaction between chlorhexidine gluconate and sodium lauryl sulfate in toothpaste reduces the effect of the mouthwash.

Chlorhexidine gluconate usage
Chlorhexidine gluconate should be used:

- Where plaque control is inadequate or difficult after surgery.
- In cases of recurrent ulceration.
- As an adjunct for periodontal therapy, for mentally or physically disabled, or medically-compromised patients.

Side effects of chlorhexidine gluconate usage
Side effects of using chlorhexidine gluconate include:

- Black/brown staining of the hard and soft tissues of the mouth, including fillings and oral appliances (dentures, removable orthodontic appliances, bite raisers etc). If it does not stain, it is not working, or the patient is not using it correctly. Gel form should be broken up and foamed around the mouth to have an effect.
- Loss of taste or changes in taste.
- Dryness and a sensation of burning of the oral mucosa [3].
- Increase in calculus formation [3].
- Parotid swelling – rare.
- Allergic reaction – this is becoming more commonly reported, and patients should be warned to stop immediately if they suspect a reaction, and contact their dentist.

Delmopinol mouthwash
Delmopinol (e.g. Decapinol®) is an effective anti-plaque/gingivitis mouthwash. Its effects are similar to chlorhexidine, but with fewer side effects, and although it can cause some staining, this is typically less than chlorhexidine and is removed with toothbrushing.

Essential oil mouthwash
Essential oil mouthwash (e.g. Listerine®) has been shown to be as effective as fluoride at reducing plaque/bacteria in the oral cavity. It can be used as a maintenance mouthwash after periodontal treatment, and is useful for patients who need an agent to maintain their gingival health without staining. However, it can cause staining.

Fluoride mouthwashes (see Chapter 11)
In addition to its remineralising ability, fluoride has certain anti-bacterial properties and is found in varying amounts in most rinses.

Several fluoride mouthwashes have been shown to reduce caries by 25–50% [2]. They can be used either once daily with a 0.05% sodium fluoride solution or once weekly by rinsing with 0.2% sodium fluoride solution. In both cases, a 10 mL solution should be rinsed around the oral cavity for 1 minute.

Fluoride mouthwash usage

Fluoride mouthwashes are particularly useful for:

- Prevention of caries in high-risk patients.
- Patients undergoing orthodontic therapy.
- Preventing root caries in older people.
- Patients with sensitive teeth.

Hydrogen peroxide mouthwashes

Hydrogen peroxide mouthwashes (e.g. Colgate® Peroxyl®) produce an oxygenated environment which hinders the function of anaerobic bacteria. They should be used for no more than 7 days at one time, and for the initial treatment of necrotising ulcerative gingivitis (see Chapter 4) and pericoronitis around partially erupted wisdom teeth.

Sodium bicarbonate

This has a neutralizing effect on acid. When dentifrices first became available early in the twentieth century, they were very expensive and people relied upon salt, bicarbonate of soda and even soot to clean their teeth. A sodium bicarbonate mouthwash can be used to quickly restore the pH of the mouth to normal after vomiting.

Benzydamine hydrochloride

Benzydamine hydrochloride (0.15% concentration) comes in either mouthwash or spray form, and is often prescribed to patients following radiotherapy for pain relief and inflammation of the throat and mouth. In mouthwash form, 15 mL should be rinsed every 1.5–3.0 hours, for no more than 7 days unless under medical supervision.

Cetylpyridinium chloride

Cetylpyridinium chloride (CPC) is found in many mouthwashes, and studies have found it to have significant anti-plaque and anti-gingivitis effects [4]. It does not work in the presence of toothpaste, and so it should be used at a different time. It can cause interproximal staining.

Sugar-free chewing gum

Sugar-free chewing gum has the following benefits:

- Increases salivary flow to wash away debris.
- Raises the pH of plaque.
- Gum containing xylitol can help inhibit the reproduction of *Streptococcus mutans* and so reduce caries rates (see Chapter 10).

ANTI-PLAQUE AGENTS

REFERENCES

1. Levine, R.S. & Stillman, C.R. (2009) *The Scientific Basis of Oral Health Education*, 6th edn. British Dental Journal, London.
2. Collins, W.J., Walsh, T. & Figures, K. (1999) *A Handbook for Dental Hygienists*, 4th edn. Butterworth Heinemann, Oxford.
3. Wilson, N., Patel, R., Gallagher, J. & Chapple, I. (2014) Dryness and a sensation of burning of the oral mucosa. *The Pharmaceutical Journal* 292, 7795.
4. Rösing, C.K., Cavagni, J., Gaio, E.J., et al. (2017) Efficacy of two mouthwashes with cetylpyridinium chloride: a controlled randomized clinical trial. *Brazilian Oral Research* 3, e47.

ANTI-PLAQUE AGENTS

Section 4

Delivering Oral Health Messages

INTRODUCTION

This section is concerned with how the oral health educator (OHE) can effectively communicate the messages learned in the preceding sections to patients and groups.

It examines the OHE's role as a communicator, including breaking down communication barriers and the basic principles of education. There is advice on setting up a preventive dental unit (PDU), obtaining or making resources for use in delivering messages, and how to plan and prepare for oral hygiene sessions and exhibitions both inside and outside the workplace. Giving practical oral hygiene instruction (OHI) is also addressed.

An OHE, like other dental care professionals (DCPs), should understand that anything they teach a patient or information given must be backed up by evidence-based scientific research, and should not be anecdotal.

Chapter 15

Communication

Learning outcomes

By the end of this chapter you should be able to:

1. Define *communication* and quote the *three rules of communication*.
2. Describe the aspects of effective communication.
3. Recognise and break down communication barriers.
4. Define *paralinguistic communication* and *neuro-linguistic programming* (NLP).
5. Recognise the role of the media and technology in patient communication.

WHAT IS COMMUNICATION?

For the oral health educator (OHE), communication involves sending information to a patient in a way that they can easily understand, remember, and act upon. It is vital that patients receive the same message that is sent.

Being able to communicate messages to a variety of patients (some of whom want to hear it, and others who do not!) is tantamount to success for the OHE, as is breaking down any communication barriers that may exist.

Most patients will have experienced occasions on leaving the surgery of a doctor, dentist, or other health professional feeling annoyed, confused, or even more nervous than when they arrived. The onus to put the patient at ease, answer questions truthfully and explain points positively, clearly, and concisely lies with the professional. It is not the patient's fault if a message is not understood. It is therefore important for the OHE to know a little communication theory.

Basic Guide to Oral Health Education and Promotion, Third Edition.
Alison Chapman and Simon H. Felton.
© 2021 John Wiley & Sons Ltd. Published 2021 by John Wiley & Sons Ltd.
Companion website: www.wiley.com/go/felton/oralhealth

The three rules of communication

The three rules of communication are:
Tell me...I forget.
Show me...I remember.
Involve me...I learn.

COMMUNICATION IN THE DENTAL SURGERY

As mentioned, the responsibility for good communication lies with the professional and forms the basis of a good relationship between the OHE and patient.

It is normal to feel nervous and apprehensive when talking to a patient. However, once you have talked to the person, found out a little about them, and planned what steps are required, the second visit (or patient) will not be nearly as intimidating. Remember that the patient may be more nervous than you are, and they are there because they need your knowledge and help.

Communication takes place at two levels:

1. Cognitive (understanding) – getting the oral health message across.
2. Emotional (related to feelings) – how the message is conveyed.

In a dental situation, the latter is often more important.

Effective communication

Effective communication makes it easier for patients to discuss problems in a relaxed, unrushed way in order to devise solutions. It should be a positive, non-threatening, unpatronising experience, which facilitates message delivery and behavioural change.

Always greet patients warmly, introducing yourself with a smile, and invite them to remove outdoor clothing and take a seat (preferably in a comfortable chair in a setting free of dental equipment, noises and smells). However, this is not always possible, and most hygienists and therapists carry out their sessions along with their clinical work, often with the patient in the dental chair. It is the educator's attitude, body language, and knowledge that put the patient at ease and helps achieve the desired results.

Advice should be clear, concise, evidence-based and consistent with health messages given by other health professionals. OHEs should use open questions, be encouraging, and tailor messages to the individual's circumstances [1].

There are three main aspects of effective (or *facilitative*) communication that the OHE should practise:

- Warmth.
- Empathy.
- Respect.

COMMUNICATION

Warmth

Warmth demonstrates interest and concern for the patient. Warmth is communicated primarily through non-verbal behaviour (i.e. active listening), such as:

- Eye contact (particularly important).
- Head nodding and body posturing (e.g. open arms not crossed).
- Facial expressions (e.g. smiling).
- Other non-verbal signs of interest and attention.

So, for example, poor non-verbal behaviour would include crossing arms and legs, and turned away from the patient, or standing above them in a menacing position (Figure 15.1). Good non-verbal behaviour would include sitting or squatting, while facing the patient, leaning forwards gently, with legs uncrossed, nodding and smiling at their level (Figure 15.2).

Empathy

Empathy means perceiving and understanding a situation from the viewpoint of another. For the OHE, it is the most important characteristic of facilitative communication. Empathy conveys the message: *I care enough to try to understand your feelings and point of view.*

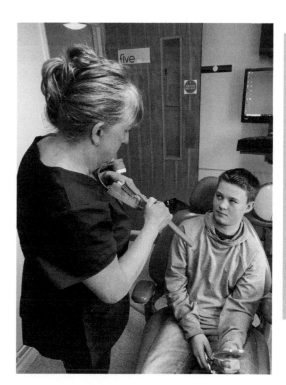

Figure 15.1 An example of poor non-verbal behaviour. Source: Simon Felton.

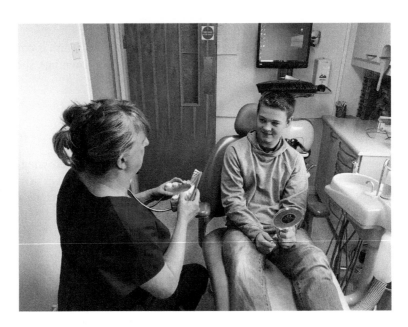

Figure 15.2 An example of good non-verbal behaviour. Source: Simon Felton.

Respect

Respect is an awareness that patients are entitled to have their own feelings, perspectives and expectations, and make decisions on their oral health treatment and management that may differ from those of the professional.

Respect does not necessarily imply agreement. It also involves taking into account issues that relate to diversity and equality. Care about your patients, be nice to them, and hopefully they will try to do anything that is asked of them.

Communication barriers

By recognising, addressing, and overcoming the following barriers by using effective communication in the surgery or when outside of the practice (e.g. giving talks, see Chapter 18), the professional will be able to engage better with individual patients.

Social/cultural barriers

There may be a social or cultural gap between the educator and patient.
   Barriers include:

- Social class (identified by dress, language, accent).
- Cultural/religious beliefs (e.g. hygiene, nutrition).

COMMUNICATION

- Language (patients that do not speak/understand or have little knowledge of English).
- Age/sex.

Limited receptiveness of patient

The OHE may want to communicate with the patient, but not the reverse. Certain patients may be unreceptive to the health professional for reasons, including:

- Mental health conditions (e.g. dementia, see Chapter 23) or confusion.
- Illness, tiredness, or pain.
- Anxiety and fear.
- Busy or distracted.
- Low self-esteem (not valuing themselves or their health).
- Not being interested in keeping healthy or looking after their teeth.

Negative attitude towards the OHE

Some patients may be *anti* the educator even before they have met because:

- Of a previous bad experience.
- They never trust people in authority.
- They see the educator as a threat (someone who will criticise or judge).
- An OHE's example conflicts with advice (e.g. educator with halitosis).
- The patient believes they know it *all* already.
- Patient has a subconscious wish not to know (e.g. results of medical tests).

Limited understanding or poor memory

Patients may have difficulties because:

- Of limited intelligence/lack of education/illiteracy.
- OHE uses jargon.
- Poor memory (cannot remember advice).
- Dementia (see Chapter 23).

Insufficient emphasis on education by the professional

Communication may fail because the professional does not put sufficient emphasis on improving skills/hygiene.

This may be because:

- It is discouraged/given low priority in their practice.
- Of a lack of confidence in the educator's own skills and knowledge.
- Inadequate training/failure to keep up to date.
- Hurried approach (not enough time allowed).

COMMUNICATION

Contradictory messages

Confusion can arise when patients receive different messages from other health professionals and acquaintances, such as:

- Dentists.
- Doctors and health visitors.
- Well-meaning family and friends.

Confusion and misunderstandings can also occur when some experts alter their views as knowledge improves and/or advice and policy changes, but not all professionals are up-to-date with such changes.

Information fade

Barriers to effective communication can lead to *information fade*, and many patients come away having remembered very little. It is therefore useful to reinforce the information given by giving a patient a leaflet to take away. Leaflets on many topics can be obtained from the representatives of dental companies or from health promotion units. OHEs can also design their own leaflets.

Paralinguistic communication

Paralinguistic communication encompasses how the manner of speech, i.e. pitch, volume, and intonation (the rise and fall of voice) is used to communicate. In other words, the manner in which words are spoken.

It can be a useful tool for the OHE in gauging the interest level of a patient, as to whether they are listening and receptive, or otherwise.

For example, the OHE should be aware that a patient who speaks in an aggressive manner may actually be hiding their fear of the dental setting, or the same words said in a hesitant tone of voice might convey disapproval and a lack of interest.

Neuro-linguistic programming training

Neuro-linguistic programming (NLP) is a way of changing someone's thoughts and behaviours to help achieve desired outcomes for them. Its uses include treatment of phobias and anxiety disorders, and improvement of workplace performance or personal happiness.

For the OHE, it can be used to formulate rapport-building techniques with the patient, so that both the OHE and the patient are on the same wavelength in order to achieve a positive outcome in improving the oral health.

Neuro-linguistic programming is a specialist subject and requires professional training. Those OHEs that are interested in acquiring NLP skills would need to attend a recognised training programme. Researching the Internet would be a good first step for those wanting to find out more.

COMMUNICATION

MEDIA INFLUENCE

Many patients and health professionals are influenced by information sourced from:

- The Internet.
- Social media platforms (e.g. Facebook, Twitter, and Instagram).
- Newspaper articles, advertising campaigns in magazines.
- TV and radio (including documentaries).

Patients will often ask the OHE about the merits of different oral health products that they have seen or heard about on these media. It is important that the OHE keeps up to date with the latest oral health products and developments within the profession by reading journals related to oral health and dental nursing (see Chapter 33), as well as keeping an eye out for product adverts, articles, and trending topics on social media. This should also be part of the OHE's continuing professional development (CPD).

If the professional can show that they have also seen a particular programme, advert, article, or trending topic that the patient is talking about, and be able to talk around the subject, the patient is more likely to respect their views on a subject that they have brought up, and respond to the OHE's advice.

The OHE can also point to recent findings that they have come across in relation to an oral health problem they are dealing with, to show that they are up to date with current thinking and developments (see Chapter 33).

TECHNOLOGY AND ORAL HEALTH EDUCATION

Technology may be of use in improving oral health in the following ways:

- Providing information and demonstrating techniques on screens for patients in the waiting room/PDU.
- The Internet is a particularly useful resource for the OHE, and certain websites can also be recommended to patients. However, be careful which websites you use/recommend, as there is plenty of good information out there, but also plenty that is erroneous. It is best to stick to recognised organisations, like those websites that come under the umbrellas of professional bodies, such as the NHS, Public Health England, the Department of Health, and the Oral Health Foundation.
- Certain oral health apps (e.g. *Sugar Smart*) can be recommended to patients, so that they can help with their own oral health (particularly relevant to young people).

COMMUNICATION

- Design software programs for producing materials for student projects as well as resources to be used with patients, including:
  - Displays and posters for use in exhibitions (see Chapter 18).
  - Leaflets for patients.

REFERENCE

1. Public Health England and Department of Health (2017) *Delivering better oral health: an evidence-based toolkit for prevention*. Available at: www.gov.uk/government/publications/delivering-better-oral-health-an-evidence-based-toolkit-for-prevention [accessed 30 April 2019].

COMMUNICATION

Chapter 16

Education and planning sessions

Learning outcomes

By the end of this chapter you should be able to:
1. Recall the works of educational theorists.
2. List and describe the *three domains of learning*.
3. Define *aims* and *objectives*.
4. Construct a lesson plan.
5. Evaluate a lesson (including questionnaires).

INTRODUCTION

When educating a patient, oral health educators (OHEs) pass on their expertise as well as their own feelings about what is being taught. The patient absorbs the information and acquires new knowledge, skills, and attitudes. The information given to the patient should be based on accurate, up-to-date, evidence-based research, rather than hearsay.

Teaching does not just happen. It has to be learned and planned meticulously, and takes plenty of practice. Before OHEs can teach or pass on knowledge, they need the basic skills to do so, i.e. the principles of education.

EDUCATIONAL THEORISTS

Education is based on theories formulated over many years by eminent academics, and the OHE should have a basic awareness of the theories of Tones and Tannahill (two expert educationalists).

Basic Guide to Oral Health Education and Promotion, Third Edition.
Alison Chapman and Simon H. Felton.
© 2021 John Wiley & Sons Ltd. Published 2021 by John Wiley & Sons Ltd.
Companion website: www.wiley.com/go/felton/oralhealth

Tones' *Model for Health Promotion* (1993) emphasised that illness is not the responsibility of the individual alone, and that many factors contribute to it, including social and environmental circumstances.

Another theorist called Tannahill produced a model of health promotion concerned with three main areas:

- Health education – educating children in healthy lifestyles.
- Health prevention – detecting problems, such as smoking or alcohol abuse.
- Heath protection – government legislation in protecting the public (e.g. drink-driving laws, and more recently smoking bans in public places).

Education experts have proved that individuals absorb what they are taught in ways related to previous experiences.

Other theorists who have developed health promotion models include *Prochaska* and *DiClemente* (see Chapter 13), Caplan and Holland (1990), Beatties (1991), and Tones and Tilford (1994). The OHE may want to look into these further for their own self-development.

THE THREE DOMAINS OF LEARNING

Before structuring a session, the OHE must decide upon which learning domain(s) their session falls into. Blinkhorn [1] described how people learn in three different ways, known as the *three domains of learning*:

1. Knowledge-related (*cognitive*). Receiving new information or explanations and thus increasing knowledge (e.g. explaining what causes caries).
2. Attitude-related. Forming and changing attitudes, beliefs, values, and opinions (e.g. a nervous patient being persuaded to visit the dentist).
3. Behaviour-related. Acquiring and improving new skills (e.g. toothbrushing).

Remember! KAB.

STRUCTURING A SESSION

After considering which domain(s) of learning a teaching session is concerned with, the OHE is ready to proceed with structuring a lesson.

However brief a session with a patient is, it is important that it is planned and structured. (While the *patient* is referred to throughout this chapter, the information is equally applicable when teaching groups, see Chapter 18.)

EDUCATION AND PLANNING SESSIONS

The stages in planning a session are:

1. Decide upon the topic.
2. Obtain background information about the patient/target group.
3. Write aims and objectives.
4. Create a lesson plan.
5. Teaching methods and aids.
6. Plan assessment and evaluation.
7. Rehearse.

Decide upon the topic

This will be either specific to an individual (related to a problem with their own oral hygiene), or relevant to a larger group, for example, talking about snacks to children. When choosing a topic, it is usually best to stick to one area, so as not to overload the audience with too much information at the same time.

Obtain background information about the patient/group

When planning an oral hygiene session, the OHE should take into consideration the following points:

- Size of audience – if too big, individual attention cannot be given.
- Prior knowledge – of the group or individual.
- Subject relevance – is the topic meeting their needs?
- Timing – too long a session leads to boredom or distraction.
- Special needs – e.g. physical or mental health conditions.
- Learning abilities – e.g. intelligence level.
- Ethnicity of groups – language/cultural barriers?
- Social class – bear in mind what products learners can afford to buy (if a requirement).

Aims

An *aim* is a statement of intent, purpose, or goal to achieve something, and is quite often general and non-specific. It should include what the patient needs to know.
Aims should be:

- Brief.
- Clear.
- Simple.
- Comprehensive – covering all the material to be taught in a session.

For example, '*I aim to teach this patient how to brush effectively*'.

Objectives

After stating the intention of the session, the next step is to plan how to achieve it. Objectives state what the patient will be able to achieve at the end of a session.

Objectives should be [1]:

- Specific (state exactly what the patient will achieve).
- Measurable (there will be a means of testing new skills, knowledge, or attitude).
- Attainable (the learning ability of the patient must be considered).
- Relevant (relating to what you want the patient to achieve).
- Time-related (what is achievable in the time available).

   Remember! SMART.

For example, by the end of the session, a patient will be able to:

- Select a suitable toothbrush for their needs.
- Carry out efficient brushing techniques.

When setting objectives, the OHE must first consider:

- The age, sex, social class, ethnicity, religion, language, and culture of the patient.
- Previous knowledge and attitudes.
- Resources available.
- Time allocated for the session.
- What the patient should realistically be able to achieve after the session.

   Words such as *know, understand* and *feel* should be avoided because they are not measurable. The OHE needs measurable objectives, using words such as: *explain, describe, state, demonstrate, discuss, select, and measure.*

   Once it is known *what* to teach, the educator must plan *how* to achieve these goals by constructing a lesson plan.

Lesson plan

All lessons, no matter how short, need a plan.

A plan enables the educator to:

- Keep to the topic.
- Refer to objectives.
- Keep to the teaching method.
- Keep to timescales.
- Assess how well the patient learned.
- Evaluate the lesson.

Table 16.1 Example lesson plan – Understanding the principles of education (*aim*).

Timing	Objectives	Subject	Method	Resources	Evaluation method
10.00 am	Introduction.	Principles of education.	Talk.	N/A.	Body language.
10.05 am	Objective 1.	Three domains of leaning.	PowerPoint® presentation.	Computer equipment.	Questions and answers.
10.15 am	Objective 2.	Aims and objectives.	PowerPoint® presentation.	Computer equipment.	Questions and answers.
10.35 am	Objective 3.	Writing aims and objectives.	Student participation.	Pens, paper.	Verbal feedback.
10.50 am	Objective 4.	Construct a lesson plan.	Group planning.	Pens, blank lesson plans.	Tutor feedback.
11.05 am	Objective 5.	Evaluation.	PowerPoint® presentation.	Computer equipment.	Answer written questions.
11.25 am	Objective 6.	Closing remarks.	Talk.	N/A.	N/A.
11.30 am	Finish.				

A lesson plan should comprise a table (e.g. Tables 16.1, 16.2), or a logical list of topics to cover.

As educators gain experience, they will refer to plans less and less. However, it is still a good idea to have a plan to double-check that nothing has been forgotten.

Table 16.2 Example lesson plan – Effective Toothbrushing using a suitable manual toothbrush (*aim*).

Timing	Objectives	Subject	Method	Resources	Evaluation method
10.00 am	Introduction.	What effective toothbrushing is and why it is important.	Talk and patient participation.	N/A.	Body language.
10.05 am	Objective 1.	Choose a suitable toothbrush.	Talk and Patient participation.	Different manual toothbrushes.	Questions and answers.
10.10 am	Objective 2.	Demonstrate an effective technique.	Talk and patient participation.	Toothbrush, plus mouth model.	Patient demonstration on model.
10.15 am	Objective 3.	Work methodically around all the teeth.	Talk and patient participation.	Toothbrush.	Patient demonstration in own mouth.
10.25 am	Objective 4.	Summarise what they have learnt, what toothbrush they need and what technique they should be using.	Talk and Q&A.	N/A.	N/A.
10.30 am	Finish.				

EDUCATION AND PLANNING SESSIONS

Teaching methods and aids

The OHE should be aware that there are many teaching methods, and that not all patients respond to the same approach. For example, some patients like to demonstrate what they have learnt back to you, others will not. Some patients remember points better if they are written down for them. Experience will gradually help the OHE plan and vary methods of teaching accordingly.

Resources and motivational aids should be relevant and simple to use/demonstrate.

Rehearse the session

It is imperative to rehearse the session using friends/family and particularly colleagues. This will help you iron out any problems and judge the amount of time needed. Be prepared to take on positive criticism and adapt your session accordingly.

Evaluation

Each teaching session needs to be evaluated.

In the context of oral health education, the term *evaluation* is used to quantify to what extent the advice given to the patient has produced tangible results. It can be defined as: *'making a judgement about the outcome and effectiveness of an oral health education session or programme'*.

Effective evaluation will tell you:

- Whether the objectives have been achieved.
- If your efforts were worthwhile.

Evaluation types

Before deciding upon evaluation methods, it is worth exploring the different types in order to select the most appropriate for a teaching session, including:

- Outcome evaluation.
- Process evaluation.
- Patient evaluation.
- Peer evaluation.
- Self-evaluation.

Outcome evaluation

What will be the outcome of the session? Will patients increase their knowledge, or change their behaviour or attitude as a result? (*Remember!* KAB.)

Process evaluation

This is concerned with session delivery as it happens. Is the teaching process going well? What is the patient telling you?

This can usually be surmised by a patient's reactions, or the signals they are giving. Observe non-verbal feedback: facial expressions and body language (see Chapter 15). Do they look interested and attentive, or are they fidgeting and looking out of the window?

From learning to spot the signs, it is possible to continually process evaluate, and adapt a session accordingly.

Patient evaluation

Take on feedback at the end of a session and be prepared to modify your teaching in future sessions.

Peer evaluation

Feedback from colleagues. Ask for comments and suggestions to improve future sessions.

Self-evaluation (reflective practice)

Look at your performance after a session. How well did it go? What worked, what did not, and why? How could the session be improved?

It is a good idea to keep a reflective practice notebook, jotting down notes about what happened immediately after each session. This enables you to identify problems and improve performance.

Evaluation methods

Having identified suitable evaluation type(s), the OHE must then select which evaluation method(s) to employ. In other words, how to assess how well a teaching session worked.

There are many methods, but whichever one(s) you choose, bear in mind that the method(s) must relate back to your aims and objectives, and show whether the goals were achieved.

Evaluation methods include:

- Question and answer session with patient. Have your questions written down in advance, so that you can refer to them in case you need to. Keep them simple, with an emphasis on getting straightforward answers. Skilful questioning will help patients give full, clear, honest answers.
- Patient demonstration of new skill – visual evaluation.
- Records of behavioural change – (e.g. plaque scores, indices, documented decrease in caries rate). This will be evaluated on return visits, after the patient has (hopefully) carried out your instructions over time. Help from the dentist or hygienist may be required here.
- Questionnaire – get the patient to fill out a questionnaire after the session (see following text).

SO WHAT IS A QUESTIONNAIRE?

A questionnaire is a relatively inexpensive and swift mechanism for collecting information or data that can be easily analysed and interpreted.

To produce a successful questionnaire, the OHE will need:

- A clear idea of an overall goal (aims and objectives).
- A good knowledge of the subject.
- Background information on the patient/target group (what are they likely to know?).
- To decide upon exactly what information needs to be answered (using *open* and *closed* questions).

Open and closed questions

There are two main types of questions in a questionnaire:

- Open questions – which provide qualitative data. For example: *'What kind of toothbrush will you use now that you have seen my exhibition?'*
- Closed questions – which provide quantitative data (Figure 16.1). For example: *'Will you now use a smaller-headed toothbrush?'*

Advantages of open questions:

- Respondents can use their own words to reply For example: *'I will use a small-headed, medium, nylon brush'*.

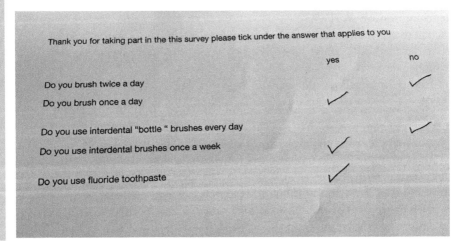

Figure 16.1 Questionnaire, closed questions. Source: Alison Chapman.

- Good when used in a pilot study as useful for finding out what people know and do not know, and can help the phrasing of questions in the final questionnaire accordingly.

Disadvantage of open questions:

- Analysis is more difficult and time-consuming to measure than closed questions.
- More time-consuming for respondent who may not answer fully.

Advantages of closed questions:

- Quick to complete – respondents just tick 'Yes' or 'No'.
- Easy analysis – questioner counts 'Yes' or 'No' answers.

Disadvantages of closed questions:

- May result in leading questions (i.e. respondents may answer as to what you lead them to write, which may not be true).
- Loss of depth – do not capture people's opinions.

Whether the educator decides to use open or closed questions (or a combination of both), care should be taken to avoid questions that are:

- Irrelevant – do not tell you what you need to know (e.g. are they male or female?).
- Offensive – make respondents feel small or embarrassed.
- Ambiguous – can be interpreted in more than one way.

It is good practice to allow respondents to remain anonymous should they wish, and a choice of opting out of answering any question they may not be comfortable with. Confidentiality is also an important consideration.

Once the type(s) of questions have been decided upon, the next stage is to design the questionnaire.

Questionnaire design

When designing a questionnaire, take into account the following considerations:

- Will a brief pilot (trial) questionnaire with a few respondents be helpful? Ask your colleagues and friends to try filling them in.
- Decide how many questions are required (10 or less if possible). People can get bored if there are too many questions, or may rush and give inaccurate responses if they are pressed for time.
- Refer back to aims and objectives to clarify the direction.
- Write questions in simple, short, easy-to-understand language.
- Give clear instructions on how to answer (e.g. *'Please tick or circle either Yes or No'*).

- If using open questions, leave sufficient space for writing answers.
- Plan how and when questionnaires will be handed out.
- Think about how they will be collected. Easy if you are there when they are completed, but notoriously difficult if people take them home – you will be very lucky to see them again! Consider using electronic questionnaires.
- Consider costs (e.g. postage).

REFERENCE

1. Blinkhorn, A.S. (2001) *Notes on Oral Health*, 5th edn. Eden Bianchi Press, Manchester.

Chapter 17
Setting up a preventive dental unit

Learning outcomes

By the end of this chapter you should be able to:
1. Describe the characteristics of a well-organised preventative dental unit (PDU).
2. Consider the factors required in setting up a PDU.
3. List the points to remember when organising a display.

INTRODUCTION

This chapter looks at the process of setting up and running a preventive dental unit (PDU) in a dental healthcare setting.

A PDU (Figure 17.1) can either be a room, self-contained area, or part of a dental surgery, where patients can be given oral health education on an informal basis in such a way that motivates them to improve their oral health. It is difficult to communicate effectively with patients during routine dental visits, and a PDU visit is ideal to focus on oral health education.

An oral health educator (OHE), with support from employers and colleagues, can develop a PDU into an integral part of the dental healthcare setting. Many patients, especially children, will look forward to their appointments and engage in improving their oral health by learning (amongst other things) about how to brush effectively, and the importance of a balanced diet.

OHEs can also get involved in other projects and displays in their workplaces, targeting issues affecting their patients and offering information on a wide range of topics. After all, the best advice for patients comes from their dental team.

Basic Guide to Oral Health Education and Promotion, Third Edition.
Alison Chapman and Simon H. Felton.
© 2021 John Wiley & Sons Ltd. Published 2021 by John Wiley & Sons Ltd.
Companion website: www.wiley.com/go/felton/oralhealth

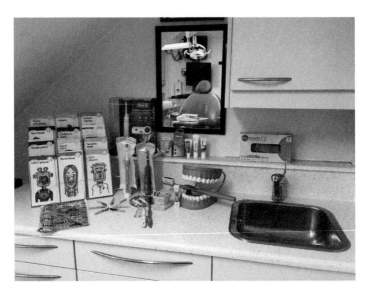

Figure 17.1 A preventive dental unit (PDU). Source: Elizabeth Hill. Reproduced with permission of Elizabeth Hill.

SETTING UP A PDU

Setting up a PDU takes a great deal of planning, care, and consultation. It is wise to ask colleagues for their thoughts and draw upon their expertise; a questionnaire is a good way to gauge their views (see Chapter 16).

To start the process you will need:

- A suitable location.
- An agreed and realistic budget.
- An approved business and marketing plan as to how the PDU will operate.
- Enthusiasm from employers and colleagues.

A suitable location

The location of the PDU should allow easy access for all patients. This can be a spare room, an area that can be partitioned off, or a surgery. The waiting room can be also used out-of-hours. Portable PDU display cabinets are available from dental suppliers, which fold away for easy storage.

Business, marketing plan and budget

It is vital to agree with the employer on how the PDU will be run alongside the practice as a business. The role of the OHE must be discussed with the employer along with an agreement as to the terms and conditions of the employment contract to include remuneration and time for the extra responsibility [1].

A budget is also necessary, and should be sufficient to allow for a well-stocked PDU, with essential resources such as:

- Mirrors.
- Mouth models.
- Toothbrushes and interdental aids.
- Leaflets.
- Games.
- Goodie bags with stickers.
- Motivational material, such as tooth brushing charts.

Enthusiasm from employers and colleagues

A well-trained and enthusiastic OHE can prove to be a great asset to any dental practice.

A supportive dental team is also essential to the success of the PDU. Dentists need to refer their patients to the OHE for oral health education, and advertising the PDU to patients using leaflets and posters in the waiting room can generate interest in the service. Reception staff are vital in managing the OHE/PDU appointment book, and promoting the service.

Regular practice meetings with news of the PDU will help keep everyone up-to-date, involved, and interested.

PDU design

The design of the PDU needs to take into account the different age groups and needs of the patients who will attend. The following are some of the design essentials for a PDU:

- Good lighting.
- Easy level access especially for those patients with restricted mobility.
- Hardwearing washable flooring.
- Robust furnishings.
- Easily cleaned worktops
- Space for leaflet displays and resources.
- Sink.
- A large mirror that is well lit and easily accessible.
- A computer to write up and store clinical records.

SETTING UP DISPLAYS

Eye-catching, relevant displays on a wide range of oral health topics can be an effective way of helping patients gain information; either in the PDU itself, or in the waiting room, where patients have time to kill when waiting for their own appointment or when attending with a friend or family member.

Planning a display

When planning a display, there are some important points to consider and arrange, including:

- Try and make full use of the space available by using display boards where possible.
- Identify your target group and set up your display accordingly (e.g. children, wheelchair users).
- Decide how long the display will be running. Leaving it running endlessly may result in some patients losing interest.
- Produce a display that coincides with, and focuses on, a national oral health campaign such as *Oral Health Month*, or *No Smoking Day/Month*.
- Use an evaluation tool such as a simple questionnaire to see how effective the display has been (see Chapter 16).

Items to display

- Posters are a great way to display information, but can become damaged quickly, so be prepared to change them. Simple, eye-catching, and clear messages are key.
- Toys and interactive games/puzzles appropriate for teaching about oral health are a great way to get patients involved.
- Mouth models help patients understand their teeth and supporting structures. They can include crowns, bridges, orthodontic appliances, and implants.
- Many leaflets/books are available on a wide range of topics, and it is a good idea to offer one to the patients after they have looked at the display to reinforce messages. They can also be produced on practice stationary with headed paper/practice logo.
- Samples of toothbrushes, toothpastes, floss, interdental aids, and mouthwashes can be obtained from wholesale dental companies, and can be used to show patients recommended products (Figure 17.2). If the practice sells the products, then companies can be generous in supplying a good selection.
- A screen showing oral hygiene techniques can be very useful. The author has lost count of the number of times patients have watched the OHE advice running on the waiting room screen and come into receive their treatment already aware of what they should be doing! This can then be backed up by the OHE and the patient given help and guidance to try a new technique.

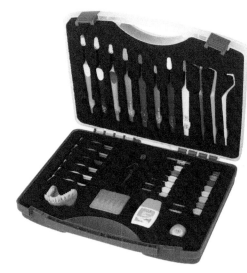

Figure 17.2 TePe® Product Presentation Case. Source: TePe Oral Hygiene Products Ltd. Reproduced with permission of TePe Oral Hygiene Products Ltd.

OTHER CONSIDERATIONS

Other important points to consider and arrange when setting up a PDU include [1]:

- Indemnity insurance for the OHE.
- An awareness of the practice's lone working protocol, and the OHE should not be isolated from the rest of the team.
- An appointment book must be established and configured to provide flexible opening times, such as after-school, school holidays, and early mornings.
- Have realistic appointment lengths to avoid keeping patients waiting, especially those with young children.
- A referral system needs to be agreed with the employer and rest of the team.
- A realistic fee scale should be agreed by the employer and rest of team.
- Accurate clinical records must be made at the time of appointment.
- A recall system for patients is useful to monitor improvements and continue motivation.
- Procedures for evaluating the service must be in place to ensure patients are able to feed back their experiences, and any improvements identified can be made.
- Compliance with GDC Standards Principle 4 (*Maintain and protect patients' information*) is essential along with GDPR (General Data Protection regulations 2018) [2].

REFERENCES

1. Hill, E. (2020) Practice Manager. Personal communication. 24th March 2020.
2. General Dental Council (2013) *Maintain and protect patients' information.* Available at: https://standards.gdc-uk.org/pages/principle4/principle4.aspx [accessed 14 December 2019].

SETTING UP A PREVENTIVE DENTAL UNIT

Chapter 18

Planning an oral hygiene presentation to a group

Learning outcomes

By the end of this chapter, you should be able to:

1. Plan a talk to a group outside of the workplace.
2. List points to consider when delivering the talk.
3. List points to consider when setting up an exhibition and a poster.

INTRODUCTION

Having covered how to construct and evaluate an oral health education session and the aspects of a PDU in which a session can be conducted with a patient, this chapter looks at practical points surrounding planning a session to a group outside of the practice, as well as designing an exhibition and a poster.

PLANNING A TALK TO A GROUP OUTSIDE OF THE PRACTICE

When planning a talk outside of the practice to a group of people, the OHE should:

1. Visit the venue in advance. On a preliminary visit check:
   - Car/disabled parking/access.
   - Public transport links.
   - Position of the room – being mindful of any medical potential conditions of attendees (e.g. room accessibility).

Basic Guide to Oral Health Education and Promotion, Third Edition.
Alison Chapman and Simon H. Felton.
© 2021 John Wiley & Sons Ltd. Published 2021 by John Wiley & Sons Ltd.
Companion website: www.wiley.com/go/felton/oralhealth

- Fire protocol and exits, and other housekeeping/safety procedures/facilities specific to the venue (and brief attendees accordingly).
- Size of the room – is it sufficient for the number of attendees?
- Lighting – bright enough?
- Electrical sockets – sufficient and in the best places for needs?
- Fixtures and fittings – are there chairs, sinks, mirrors?
- Resources available (e.g. computer, projector, screen, flipcharts, tables, chairs).
- Refreshments and facilities (e.g. kitchen, bathroom).

2. Book a date with the venue owner or organiser (obtain proof of booking where applicable), and confirm the booking nearer the time.
3. Obtain background information on the group from a group leader/ teacher/community leader, etc.
4. Work out costs – keep within a specified budget.
5. Decide upon the topic, aims and objectives, lesson plan, and evaluation (see Chapter 16).
6. Collect visual aids/resources.
7. Rehearse talk – using colleagues/friends/family. Take on board constructive criticism.

DELIVERING THE TALK (CHECKLIST)

On the actual day of the talk:

1. Check and double-check you have everything before leaving for the venue.
2. Arrive early.
3. Ensure the room is arranged as required.
4. Set out resources.
5. Welcome the audience, introduce yourself and anyone else involved in delivering the session. Go through housekeeping of venue.
6. Tell them what you are going to cover and the format/length.
7. Speak slowly and clearly so that everyone can hear – ask them!
8. Encourage group participation.
9. Use a variety of teaching methods (to avoid boredom).
10. Avoid technical jargon (unless talking to fellow professionals).
11. Encourage motivation and awareness.
12. Allow supervised practice of new skills (if applicable).
13. Reinforce learning – using handouts and/or leaflets.
14. Summarise what you have covered (*tell them what you have told them*).

15. Finish on time – people get restless if a session overruns (and have suitable breaks).
16. Arrange a return visit to follow up on learning (if possible/required).

Remember to thank the group for their attention, teachers or group/community leaders for their help, and colleagues for their support if applicable. Leave your contact details for attendees in case they have subsequent questions. Leave the venue as you found it.

SETTING UP AN EXHIBITION OR DISPLAY

Planning an exhibition or a display also requires much thought and preparation, and the following stages should be followed:

1. Decide upon the topic, aims and objectives, and target group(s).
2. Decide on the type of exhibition (e.g. notice boards, free-standing, computer programme).
3. Consider lighting and the position of the exhibition – maximise its visibility.
4. Consider the height of those who will view it.
5. Set up tables if needed.
6. Make the exhibition simple, eye-catching, and interesting.
7. Organise information in short sections under clear headings.
8. Arrange times to stay with the exhibition and talk to the public/patients.
9. Prepare and supervise an evaluation method (see Chapter 16).

POSTER DESIGN AND DISPLAYING WRITTEN INFORMATION

When planning and preparing a poster (or other written information) for an exhibition or display, the following points should be considered:

- Experiment with colour combinations (e.g. yellow on black shows up well; yellow on white is not good; red is eye-catching, but too much red may be overpowering).
- Write clearly and large enough for the information to be read easily (thick felt-tip pens work well).

- Consider word-processed material, which gives text clarity (especially for those with less neat handwriting!)
- Vary the colour and size of text for extra emphasis.
- Do not write too much, concentrate on the main message(s), and leave sufficient white space to help make your points clear.
- More detailed information can be given in the form of leaflets.

Remember! Whether planning a talk or an exhibition within the practice, or at an outside venue, use technology wisely and involve colleagues whenever possible; they often have hidden talents and good ideas.

Chapter 19

Practical oral hygiene instruction

Learning outcomes

By the end of this chapter you should be able to:
1. Motivate patients to improve plaque control.
2. Explain and carry out disclosing.
3. Advise patients on suitable toothbrushes.
4. Demonstrate toothbrushing techniques.
5. Give practical instruction on interdental and tongue cleaning.
6. Advise patients on complementary and alternative therapies.
7. Give an example of a model practical OHE appointment.

INTRODUCTION

Practical oral hygiene instruction (OHI) is a vital role of the oral health educator (OHE).

In order to gain confidence in giving instruction and practical help to patients, the OHE needs to understand the theories of tooth cleaning and continually update their knowledge on the latest techniques and methods. (Specific advice for certain target groups is covered in Section 5.)

UK law is ambiguous on whether a dental nurse can put toothbrushes and other cleaning aids in patients' mouths. A good guideline for the OHE is to have written instructions from their dentist on what they are allowed to carry out, and observe the General Dental Council's *Scope of Practice* (see Chapter 31).

In this age of litigation, the OHE must make contemporaneous notes in case a patient should ever decide that they want to make a complaint. Consent and the explanation of disease are of paramount importance and should be

Basic Guide to Oral Health Education and Promotion, Third Edition.
Alison Chapman and Simon H. Felton.
© 2021 John Wiley & Sons Ltd. Published 2021 by John Wiley & Sons Ltd.
Companion website: www.wiley.com/go/felton/oralhealth

documented. The OHE must have indemnity cover for oral hygiene instruction, and it can be included in the employer's cover or individual cover [1].

TEACHING PLAQUE CONTROL SKILLS

Research shows [2–4] that whilst effective plaque control alone has little effect on the rate of caries, it is the single most important method of preventing periodontal disease. (In the prevention of caries, other factors such as diet, fissure sealing, and fluoride are also involved.)

In practical OHI sessions, the OHE must be able to:

- Motivate patients to improve plaque control.
- Explain and demonstrate disclosing.
- Give practical instruction on interdental cleaning.
- Advise on the most suitable toothbrush for their use.
- Demonstrate suitable toothbrushing techniques.
- Discuss the advantages and disadvantages of various toothpastes.

Patient motivation

Communication skills are heavily involved in motivation, although the OHE will also need:

- Time to talk to the patient, to find out background information about them.
- A relaxed, unhurried approach.
- Empathy with patient difficulties and problems (see Chapter 15).
- Regular appointments to assess progress.
- Endless patience!

Telling someone about a problem does not motivate them to change. Giving them evidence in various formats can help:

- Use written information.
- Images of periodontal disease progression.
- Observation – disclosing or identifying areas of inflammation by looking in the mirror.
- X-rays and pocket charts.

Ask the patient what they understand and use this framework to explain the need for change. Try to limit the amount of information to no more than three instructions at each appointment. Patients who are bombarded with information and habit changes at an initial appointment are less likely to remember and act.

Set a goal for each intervention for the patient to achieve after each appointment. Explain that having a clean at the dentist removes plaque for one day, and that they are responsible for the other 364 days of the year. On average it takes 66 attempts to form a habit, so don't be too disheartened when they come back and haven't been cleaning interdentally on a daily basis [5].

Try to be positive, to help them believe they can change. Asking them to plan when they will carry out a particular oral hygiene technique can help them to undertake it. For example, when would be the best time for them to use interdental brushes? Although we know the best time to clean interdentally is before brushing at night, motivating them to do it daily will still be effective. Suggest patients put an alarm on their phone to remind them each day, for example.

Disclosing

The use of disclosing tablets or solution is a good way of enabling patients to identify fresh and mature plaque, highlighted by different colour staining (Figure 19.1). This can be combined with a plaque index (see Chapter 29) and

(a)

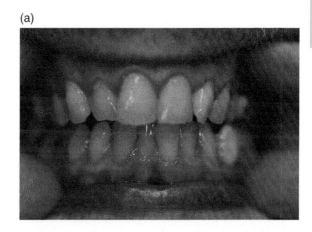

(b)

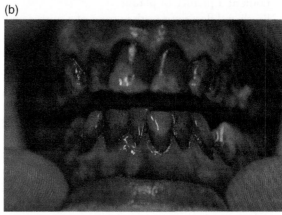

Figure 19.1 Plaque – (a) undisclosed; (b) disclosed. Source: Alison Chapman.

PRACTICAL ORAL HYGIENE INSTRUCTION

used to motivate the patient by producing a score, which the patient is encouraged to reduce by improved oral hygiene methods.

Suggest that the patient discloses:

- Regularly – perhaps once a week until plaque-removing skills improve. Get them to suggest when they would be able to do this. (Sunday is a good day for many.)
- After interdental cleaning and brushing to highlight difficult areas.
- At a suitable time of day (e.g. not when they are about to go out).

The patient should apply a thin layer of petroleum jelly to their lips to prevent staining.

There are various disclosing agents available: the common active ingredient being erythrosine (a harmless, tasteless, red food dye). Disclosing can be a fun method for encouraging children to improve their oral hygiene, and parents could take photographs to compare results as the children practise and hopefully improve their oral hygiene techniques. When advising children, you must involve the parent and explain the correct use of the tablet or solution and that it can be a messy procedure. Try giving the patient a hand mirror and asking them to point out where they can improve their oral hygiene. This involves the patient thinking about what they need to do, and identifying the areas they need to work on.

Disclosing exercises

It is a good idea to practise your own disclosing techniques using the following exercises.

Exercise 1

- Disclose your own mouth after eating a meal (of fairly sticky foods) and before brushing your teeth.
- Gently remove some plaque using floss or tape.
- Look at the plaque and try to remember what it consists of.
- Look at a picture of plaque.
- Brush and floss your teeth in front of a mirror until no trace of plaque remains.
- Disclose your mouth again, to see if you have succeeded in your own oral health procedures – you may be surprised at how difficult it is to remove plaque effectively.

Exercise 2

Now you can move on and test your skills on someone else.

- Find an obliging friend or relative who will help you check your learning.
- Put petroleum jelly on their lips (to minimise staining), then help the patient disclose the plaque.
- Explain what plaque is to your patient in simple terms that a non-dental expert would understand.

- Ask if your explanation was easy to understand.
- Take note of patient comments (i.e. patient evaluation).

Exercise 3
- Find a dentally-trained colleague.
- Using your dental knowledge and technical jargon, explain the development of plaque from the salivary pellicle stage to mature plaque.
- Ask for feedback and constructive criticism on your performance.
- Do not be offended if you were not perfect – keep practising.

Plaque indicator kits

Plaque indicator kits can be used to demonstrate the age of plaque – showing fresh and more mature deposits depending on the colour – pink/red (for fresh plaque) to blue/purple, which is at least 48 hours old.

A sample of plaque is removed and placed in a liquid, then left for 5 minutes to develop. The colour is checked against a pH chart denoting its acidity level, which could be indicative of a patient's caries susceptibility. The plaque is then exposed to a solution representing saliva to demonstrate the saliva's buffering ability.

Toothbrushes

Advise patients on a suitable choice of toothbrush. There are so many toothbrushes on the market now that it is difficult to know which one to advise. Many dental practices sell specific brands and the OHE will probably use brushes from the range stocked for demonstration purposes.

Patients may also ask about biodegradable brushes (e.g. TePe GOOD™). The OHE should keep up-to-date with this fast developing area, and be able to give an opinion as to what is available and suitable.

It is more important to ensure that patients clean their mouths effectively rather than to insist on a particular toothbrush being used.

Remember when advising on toothbrushes:

- Suggest a good quality, medium-textured brush with nylon filaments and a small enough head to suit the patient.
- Suggest a simple design (often most effective).
- Remind the patient to change a brush when filaments show signs of wear or after about 2–3 months.

Power brushes
Power brushes (also known as *electric toothbrushes*) are commonly used, and the OHE should advise a patient, when choosing a powered brush, to buy a rechargeable brush with a 2-minute timer and pressure sensor if possible.

Oscillating-rotating or sonic brushes are both effective. The head should be changed every 2–3 months, and if the bristles are bending outward they have been putting too much pressure on the brush.

Tell the patient that there is still a need for daily interdental cleaning even when using a powered brush. Oral-B®/Braun™ models have an interdental brush head, which is suitable for large gaps between teeth, to reach behind upper molars, lingually for lower molars, and tightly crowded irregular teeth.

Manual toothbrushing

Before deciding upon the most effective brushing technique for the patient, the OHE should be able to advise on a suitable choice of toothbrush. However, it is also advisable to ask the patient to bring their toothbrush, so they can practise in their own mouth.

It is important to instruct patients in a method appropriate to the size and shape of their mouths and manual dexterity, and suggest frequency of brushing, i.e. last thing at night and once in the day, preferably in the morning.

There are many different methods of toothbrushing. Some are designed to clean specific areas of the mouth, and some are more difficult to master than others. Patients should be encouraged to have a methodical approach to brushing, remembering to include the lingual and palatal surfaces.

The OHE should take into account the patient's:

- Needs – what is their plaque control like? Is gingivitis or periodontitis present?
- Time – will the patient spend time on a particular technique?
- Manual dexterity – not all patients can cope with certain techniques.

Remember! After brushing, patients should only spit the toothpaste out and not rinse it away (toothpaste in the sink will not benefit their teeth!).

Brushing techniques

Whichever of the following techniques is used, the OHE should demonstrate on a mouth model, then give the patient a brush and ask for a repeat demonstration on the model and then in their own mouth (Figure 19.2). If the patient is removing plaque effectively using their own 'style', do not try to change the toothbrushing technique. It may be a combination of some or all of the following methods but if it is effective – this does not matter!

Bass technique/modified Bass (Figure 19.3)

The toothbrush is placed with the filaments at a 45 degree angle towards the gingival crevice. A gentle, circular movement is designed to remove bacteria from the crevice, but requires considerable dexterity and not all patients can cope. In *modified Bass*, the action ends by rolling the brush down in an occlusal direction.

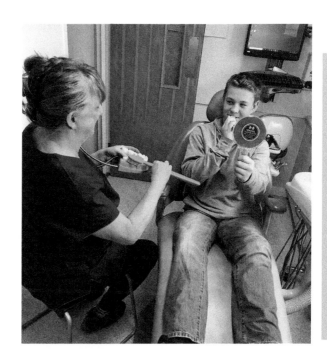

Figure 19.2 Repeating demonstration of toothbrushing. Source: Simon Felton.

Simple scrub

Similar to Bass, this is the technique recommended by the *Scientific Basis of Oral Health Education* [4]. Angle the brush towards the gingival margin and cover all surfaces using short, horizontal movements.

Fones (circular) technique (Figure 19.4)

Particularly appropriate for children as it is relatively easy and teaches them to brush the gingivae as well as teeth. The teeth are held in occlusion and large circular movements performed. The child must then be shown how to clean the lingual and occlusal surfaces with a gentle scrubbing action. With a very small child, it is a good idea to have them sit on the floor, with their back to the parent, who is sitting on a chair and holding the child between his/her knees. Tilt the chin gently upwards so that a good view is obtained and then have them perform the technique as described.

Brushing with a power brush (Figure 19.5)

Work systematically around the mouth, one tooth at a time, angling the brush so that the bristles are aimed toward the gingival margin at an angle of approximately 45 degrees, gently moving the brush along the tooth/gingival margin allowing the brush to do the work. The patient should try not to put too much pressure on the brush as this stalls it and stops it working. (Some brushes have an indicator light to show when this is happening).

(a)

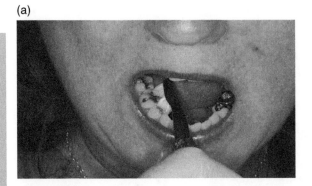

(b)

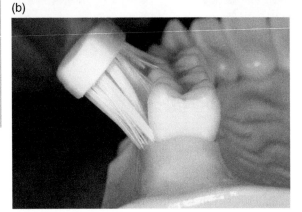

Figure 19.3 (a,b) Bass technique. Source: Dr Ian Bellamy. Reproduced with permission of Dr Ian Bellamy.

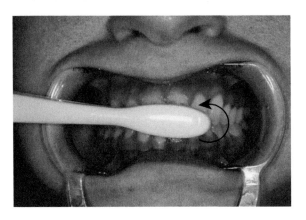

Figure 19.4 Fones (circular) technique. Source: Alison Chapman.

Be sure to take in the lingual aspects of lower molars and buccal/distal aspects of upper molars, and lingual and palatal surfaces as well. Complete the brushing by gently running the brush along occlusal surfaces.

You may suggest *breaking* their mouth into four quarters and spending 30 seconds cleaning each, which would make up the recommended 2 minutes.

(a)

(b)

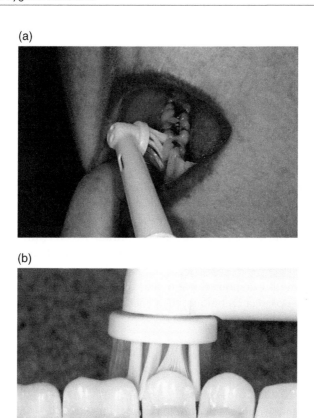

Figure 19.5 Patient demonstrating flossing skill. Source: Simon Felton. (a,b) Power brush technique. Source: Dr Ian Bellamy. Reproduced with permission of Dr Ian Bellamy.

When to brush

Brushing should be done last thing at night with nothing to eat or drink afterwards except water, and at one other time during the day.

Patients may ask if they should brush before or after breakfast. This depends on what they have for breakfast; anything acidic may slightly soften the enamel and brushing could wear this away. The buffering action of saliva will harden it after approximately one hour. (See Chapter 6, the Stephan Curve.)

Interdental cleaning methods

Most patients are well aware of the importance of toothbrushing, but many are still not cleaning interdental areas regularly, and do not realise that this is important in preventing gingivitis and periodontal disease, as well as some systemic diseases.

Patients should be taught to clean interdentally before they brush. Interdental cleaning after brushing will remove the toothpaste residue and is not to be advised (nor is using a mouthwash after brushing).

OHEs must be able to advise on the different methods available and suggest the most suitable for each patient, including floss and tape, interdental brushes, rubber toothpicks, and water irrigation units.

Floss and tape

If used effectively, floss and tape are probably the most efficient ways of removing plaque interdentally in patients who have no periodontal pocketing, or tight/overcrowded teeth.

The OHE should be aware of the different types of floss, such as waxed and unwaxed, and patients should be encouraged to try different types of floss and tape, to see which they prefer, and try a floss handle if indicated (Figure 19.6).

The OHE should demonstrate flossing on a model and show pictures or diagrams of the correct technique, then encourage the patient to demonstrate their skill (Figure 19.7).

How to use floss and tape

Follow these steps:

- Take about 20 cm of floss.
- Wrap each end around each middle finger (Figure 19.8).
- Using thumbs and index fingers to manoeuvre and keeping the floss taught, gently slide backwards and forwards between contact points.
- On reaching the gingival margin, curve the floss into a 'c' shape around the tooth surface (Figure 19.9).
- Move up and down a few millimetres under the gingival margin.
- Then take over the interdental papillae and curve around the adjacent tooth, and repeat.

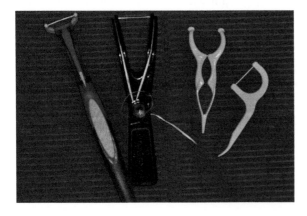

Figure 19.6 Different types of floss handles. Source: Alison Chapman.

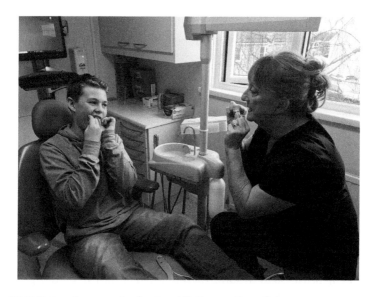

Figure 19.7 Patient demonstrating flossing skill. Source: Simon Felton.

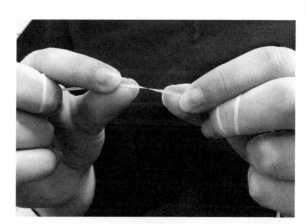

Figure 19.8 Floss usage (wrapped around fingers). Source: Alison Chapman.

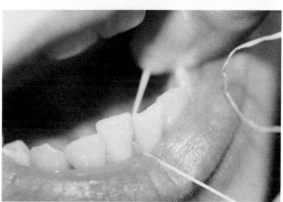

Figure 19.9 Interdental plaque removal (using floss). Source: Carole Hollins. Reproduced with permission of Carole Hollins.

- Make floss taught again and gently slide backwards and forwards to remove from the interdental area.
- Repeat between teeth.

If the patient finds this difficult, they can be taught to tie a loop with the floss, put all their fingers in the loop then continue as before (Figure 19.10). Floss handles and floss picks can make this process much easier and should be considered when teaching children to floss (see Chapter 21).

Interdental brushes

Interdental brushes (Figure 19.11) are most effective for patients who have pocketing or bone loss.

When using a brush, the tip should be placed at the gingival margin and a back and forth twisting action used to insert between the teeth. The brush should be moved in and out between the teeth 5–10 times before moving onto the next interdental space. Patients should be made aware that they would need different brush sizes around the mouth. The brush should go through with some resistance in order to disturb the plaque.

For patients with advanced periodontal disease, there are many different brushes available, and the OHE should be aware of the designs, which can aid access.

Rubber toothpicks (Figure 19.12)

These can be useful for smaller spaces and for patients who cannot manage interdental brushes. Patients may start off using these then move on to interdental brushes as they become more skilled.

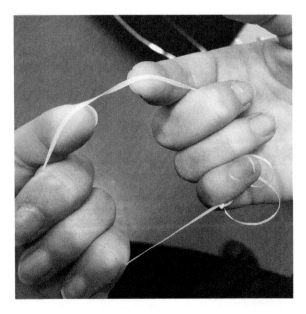

Figure 19.10 Floss usage (fingers in loop). Source: Alison Chapman.

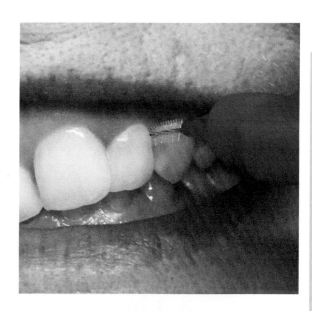

Figure 19.11 Interdental brush usage. Source: Alison Chapman.

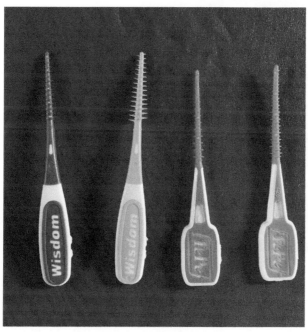

Figure 19.12 Rubber toothpicks. Source: Alison Chapman.

Interspace brushes (Figure 19.13)

These handy little brushes have many uses, including around implants, over-crowded or instanding teeth and behind those difficult to reach, including the

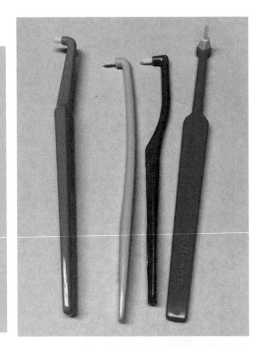

Figure 19.13 Interspace brushes.
Source: Alison Chapman.

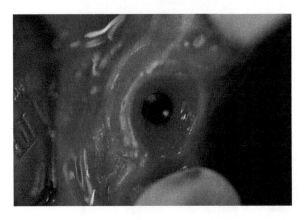

Figure 19.14 Gingival
sulcus depth, implant. Source:
Alison Chapman.

back molars. They can also be useful where patients have a strong gag reflex or
in larger spaces between teeth. Patients with periodontal disease can be taught
to use them around each individual tooth, taking their fine tip right down into
the pocket and sweeping around the root to disturb the biofilm.

Implant, braces, and bridge cleaning

There are many different implant designs, which should all be cleaned using a
normal brushing technique, but because the gingival crevice is much deeper with
implants (Figure 19.14), patients should also be instructed to use an interspace

brush, wiping it around the implant to enter the crevice. Alternatively, use Tepe® Bridge and Implant Floss/Oral B Superfloss™ (wrapped around the implant, crossed over and sawed back and forth entering the crevice).

Implants

Implants that form part of a bridge may also need bridge and implant floss to clean around them. This floss has a stiffened end to pass under the bridge and a thicker section to clean under the bridge. It can also be used to clean abutments by curving and wiping up and down the abutment.

Bridges

For bridges, interdental brushes can be used to clean the abutment areas. Bridge and implant floss (Figure 19.15) can be used to thread under the bridge and eased along it to remove debris from underneath the bridge and clean to the abutment.

Fixed braces

These should be cleaned with a toothbrush (manual or powered). Clean along the gingival margin as normal, then again along the wires, aiming the bristles towards the wire. Interdental brushes or an interspace brush can be used to clean around the brackets.

Water irrigation units

Water irrigation units can help to remove food debris and some plaque from interdental spaces. They use a pressured jet of water or mouthwash to pass between the teeth. However, they cannot expand and contract to fill the whole space, so they are not as effective as interdental brushes.

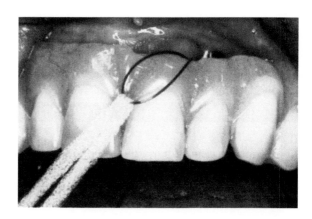

Figure 19.15 Floss threader on a fixed bridge. Source: Mary Mowbray. Reproduced with permission of Mary Mowbray.

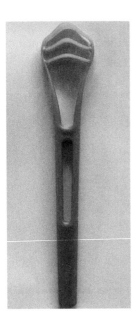

Figure 19.16 Tongue scraper. Source: Alison Chapman.

Tongue cleaning

Bacteria on the tongue can contribute to bad breath (as well as bacteria found on teeth and interdentally), and a tongue scraper (Figure 19.16) can be used to help this condition and freshen the mouth.

The tongue cleaner should be placed towards the back of the tongue and brushed/dragged forwards across the surface. Alternatively, the patient my use their toothbrush to do this.

Advice to orthodontic appliance wearers

For advice on cleaning orthodontic appliances see Chapter 22.

Advice to denture wearers

For advice on cleaning dentures see Chapter 23.

COMPLEMENTARY AND ALTERNATIVE THERAPIES

Complementary and alternative therapies have been used for thousands of years, long before the advent of conventional medicine. They range from homeopathy, aromatherapy and herbalism using plant material; acupuncture to stimulate the network of energy patterns that runs through the body; osteopathy, and hypnosis.

With some patients now taking a holistic (*whole body*) approach to health, the OHE should be aware of these other forms of therapy. Patients have a right to choose what treatment they undertake and this should be respected. For example, some patients think that fluoride is a poison and consequently do not use fluoride toothpastes. It is their right to choose and while the OHE might like to discuss their opinions, one should also respect their right and be prepared to advise accordingly – for example, that the patient reduces sugar frequency and applies effective oral hygiene techniques.

OHEs work under the prescription of a dentist, and even if they are knowledgeable in complementary and alternative therapies, they may only use these therapies when practising if specifically qualified to do so, and if the dentist has prescribed the treatment.

Acupuncture

Acupuncture is used to relieve:

- Gagging.
- Nausea.
- Temporomandibular joint (TMJ) pain and muscle disorders.
- Headaches and other pain.

Herbal remedies

Herbal remedies include:

- Echinacea – a healing promoter, with additional antimicrobial, anti-inflammatory, and analgesic properties. Can be used in the treatment of periodontal disease.
- Sanguinarine – found in some mouthwashes and toothpastes. It kills bacteria (helping reduce dental caries) and has anti-inflammatory effects (apparently helping to reduce gingivitis). This is no longer used in dental products as it increases the risk of developing leukoplakia, which can become cancerous (see Chapter 8).
- Aloe vera – antibacterial qualities. Can be found in toothpastes, and can help with ailments such as angular cheilitis (see Chapter 8). It is thought to stimulate the immune system, is a mild antiseptic and can be used as a mouthwash, which does not sting (e.g. Weleda).
- Chinese herbs – can be used for treating periodontal disease.

Aromatherapy

Forms of aromatherapy include:

- Lavender – calming effect; can be used in reception or the surgery to help anxious patients.
- Tea tree oil – an antimicrobial used topically to treat minor skin conditions, such as acne or sore throats. It can be toxic if overused in the oral cavity.

Homeopathy

Forms of homeopathy include:

- Arnica – for bruising, trauma, shock, and any dental procedures.
- Hypericum – for injured nerves, e.g. root canal treatment (RCT).
- Aconite – for fear and anxiety.
- Chamomilla – for teething.
- Feverfew – for aphthous ulcers.
- Propolis ointment – for aphthous ulcers, lichen planus, angular cheilitis, cracked lips, and cold sores (see Chapter 8).

EXAMPLE OHE APPOINTMENT [1]

The following scenario takes you through the steps taken in a practical OHI session, including record keeping (in *italics*). In this case, the patient (a junior school child) has been referred to you (an OHE) regarding their oral health.

Action: You prepare for their visit by checking on their patient record to give you an idea of what to expect, which reads: *Pt ref by GDP for OHE re: poor plaque control, early single/multiple caries developed, advice on diet.*

Action: You introduce yourself to the child and their mum who has also attended, by telling them your name and that you are a dental nurse who has had special training to talk to children and adults about looking after their teeth at home. You confirm the patient's medical history with the parent and say that their dentist has asked if they could visit to talk about the reason why they have been referred to you.

Action: You then ask them (and their mum), if you can have a look inside their mouth, and you have a look at their oral cavity with your gloves and mask on (Figure 19.17). You then take those off and sit by them on the dental stool in an open, friendly way (see Chapter 15).

You write on their record: *Pt attended with mum. Pt's medical history and oral hygiene regime checked.* If no relevant medical history, you write *NRMH*

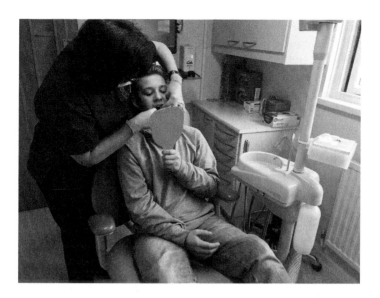

Figure 19.17 OHE looking inside patient's mouth. Source: Simon Felton.

(no relevant medical history). If something is contraindicated, then you write this in the notes to acknowledge it. You establish that the patient, *Uses a manual toothbrush (mtb) 2 x daily with fluoride toothpaste (ftp), no mouthwash used. No other OH aids used.*

Action: You then ask the patient to demonstrate their toothbrushing method.

You write on their record: *OHI/TBI. I asked pt to demonstrate their tb method on mouth model to see how they tb at home.* You write what they actually do, e.g. *tb 1 x daily for 30 seconds.*

Action: You then ask how long do they think they brush for, and if they rinse their mouth out after brushing. You demonstrate the circular/scrub technique on a mouth model, using a timer to demonstrate 2 minutes (which may surprise them). Then you ask them to demonstrate the same technique to see if their technique has improved.

You write on their record: *Demonstrated circular/scrub on mouth model for 2 mins and pt demonstrated technique again, which improved.*

Action: You then ask permission to disclose their mouth (using petroleum jelly on their lips and a bib to protect their clothes).

Action: They stand at the sink to brush their teeth after seeing the results in a handheld mirror. They either use their own toothbrush or you give them a suitably sized new one. The results after toothbrushing are checked in the mirror and you ask them if their teeth feel cleaner and silky? They usually say they do. You tell them to use adult toothpaste and brush the way they just did for 2 minutes twice a day, ideally once in the morning and once last thing at night. You explain this helps the toothpaste protect their teeth for longer.

You write on their record: *Disclosed pt's mouth and they checked their brushing. Rx (Recommended with good luck!) to tb 2 x daily for 2 minutes with an adult ftp and to spit out not rinse out after tb.*

Action: You then briefly explain plaque formation in very simple terms and the importance of brushing it away regularly to have healthy teeth and gums.

Action: For their diet, you go through their likes and dislikes and what they eat on a daily basis. Then you test them on how many teaspoons of sugar are in certain foods/drinks, and they are usually surprised by the amounts. You recommend the *Sugar Smart* app if they (or their parent) has a smart phone. They can check the sugar content in many foods and drinks just by scanning the bar codes. You advise them to limit the frequency of sugar intake to meal-times only.

You write on their record: *Discussed diet, recommended sugar intake, Sugar Smart app. Highlighted high sugar foods and drinks and advised to limit the frequency of sugar intake to mealtimes only.* (If patient has high caries rate maybe suggest a diet diary for 3 days.)

Action: You give them a sample of toothpaste, tell them they can keep their new brush, plus they get a goodie bag and a diet sheet with recommended foods and drinks, a tooth brushing chart, a new pencil, and a leaflet on brushing and sugars in foods.

Action: Finally, you ask them if they have any questions and answer them as best you can, and also ask if they have found the session useful. A review appointment is sometimes made, but if they are seeing their dentist soon, then you ask the dentist to review at next visit.

REFERENCES

1. Hill, E. (2020) Practice Manager. Personal communication. 20th January 2020.
2. Fejerskov, O. & Kidd, E. (2004) *Dental Caries: The Disease and Its Clinical Management*. Blackwell Munksgaard, Oxford.
3. Lindhe, J., Karring, T. & Lang, N. (2003) *Clinical Periodontology and Implant Dentistry*, 4th edn. Blackwell Munksgaard, Oxford.
4. Levine, R.S. & Stillman, C.R. (2009) *The Scientific Basis of Oral Health Education*, 6th edn. British Dental Journal, London.
5. Lally, P., Cornelia, H., van Jaarsveld, M., *et al.* (2009) How are habits formed: Modelling habit formation in the real world. European Journal of Social Psychology 40, 998–1009.

Section 5

Oral Health Target Groups and Case Studies

INTRODUCTION

This section explores delivering oral health education to at-risk target groups.

Although all patients should be given advice regarding general and dental health, for those patients with whom there is a greater concern, special attention needs to be applied. It is vital that all members of the dental team and other health care workers give the same advice to these groups.

The section details particular problems, which may be encountered when dealing with patients who need specialised care and attention from dental professionals for a number of reasons. It concludes with a chapter on carrying out case studies, which will be particularly useful for dental nurses studying for an oral health education qualification.

Chapter 20

Pregnant patients

Learning outcomes

By the end of this chapter you should be able to:

1. Discuss dental issues and conditions related to pregnancy with patients.
2. List the signs and symptoms of pregnancy gingivitis.
3. Advise patients on lifestyle and risks (including smoking, diet, and alcohol).

INTRODUCTION

Pregnant women are an important target group. Good advice on the oral cavity during pregnancy is essential as pregnant patients have an increased risk of gingival damage, caries and tooth erosion. Diet, alcohol, and smoking (see Chapters 9 and 13) are also important factors for the oral and general health of the patient and the unborn child.

The oral health educator (OHE) should be able to explain changes that pregnant mothers may have noticed in the health of their mouths, give advice and reassurance, and help them develop an effective oral health routine, which they can continue as their family grows. The OHE should also be able to provide basic advice (and *signposting*) on diet and lifestyle.

Pregnant women are generally very receptive to information and keen to do the best they can for their health and that of the coming baby. During routine antenatal care, they are encouraged to seek dental advice, and many who are not regular dental attendees, will attend during pregnancy for the sake of their coming child. They are encouraged further in the UK as NHS practices offer free treatment to pregnant women, although it is often difficult to register with an NHS practice and many pregnant patients therefore opt to stay with their private practice.

Basic Guide to Oral Health Education and Promotion, Third Edition.
Alison Chapman and Simon H. Felton.
© 2021 John Wiley & Sons Ltd. Published 2021 by John Wiley & Sons Ltd.
Companion website: www.wiley.com/go/felton/oralhealth

Also, some pregnant patients (particularly in socially-deprived areas) are unaware of the need for good oral hygiene and diet during pregnancy.

Lifestyle advice during pregnancy

It is important not to give out-of-date or conflicting advice, and OHEs should check what guidance other members of the healthcare team (e.g. midwives) are giving to pregnant women.

Be aware of local and national initiatives, such as *Start4life* in England – an NHS programme which gives good advice on diet and lifestyle for pregnant patients [1]. In Scotland, *Ready Steady Baby*, and, in Wales, *Your Pregnancy and Baby Guide* are also excellent resources [2,3].

Questions on the developing embryo and foetus

The OHE should be able to explain how the oral cavity develops in the growing embryo and foetus in case a patient asks, particularly with reference to queries about cleft lip and palate (see Chapter 1).

SUSCEPTIBILITY TO ORAL DISEASES AND CONDITIONS

A patient's susceptibility to the following oral diseases and conditions can increase during pregnancy.

Erosion (see also Chapter 6)

Susceptibility to erosion can increase during pregnancy due to:

* Vomiting (morning sickness) – regurgitation of stomach acids.
* Acid reflux, heartburn – stomach acid passes into the oesophagus and mouth.
* Increased acidic foods/drinks intake. An increased intake of healthier foods by pregnant women may inadvertently increase acidic drinks and foods, such as fruit, fruit juices, and dressed salads.

Prevention/management

Provide advice on:

* Diet. Restricting acidic foods and drinks (and limit to regular mealtimes).
* Gentle toothbrushing – allow an hour after consuming acidic foods or drinks. Do not brush immediately after vomiting.
* Fluoride application – to increase tooth resistance to acid (e.g. toothpaste, mouthwash).

Caries (see Chapter 5)

Susceptibility to caries can increase during pregnancy, due to:

- Cravings/frequent snacking (often for sweet foods).
- Nausea when toothbrushing and/or a dislike of the taste of a particular toothpaste, which can lead to less frequent toothbrushing.

Prevention/management
Provide advice on:

- Diet/sugar-free snacks/smoking (see Chapters 9, 10 and 13).
- Alternative toothpastes – that have a more acceptable flavour (see Chapter 14).

Gingival problems (see Chapter 3)

An increased risk of gingival problems in pregnant patients is due to:

- Nausea – preventing effective oral hygiene, usually in the early weeks, but may continue throughout pregnancy.
- Hormonal changes – causing an exaggerated response to plaque toxins.

Pregnancy gingivitis
Pregnancy gingivitis is a common problem, which results from hormonal changes that increase blood supply during pregnancy to ensure that the growing baby is constantly provided with the nutrients it needs to develop and grow. The downside being that increased blood flow can cause gums to swell and sometimes bleed.

This worrying and sometimes uncomfortable condition usually resolves itself once the baby is born. However, if untreated, it can lead to permanent damage to the periodontium. Pregnancy gingivitis is more likely to occur in women who have poor oral hygiene and/or gingival problems before pregnancy, but it can also affect women with excellent oral hygiene and previously healthy gums. There is also an exaggerated response to dental plaque due to increased hormone activity.

Symptoms of pregnancy gingivitis
The patient may complain of:

- Bleeding on brushing – sometimes profuse and where none has occurred before.
- Spontaneous bleeding – blood on the pillow or when eating crisp foods (e.g. apple).
- Occasional irritation or itchiness of the gums.
- Halitosis.

Signs of pregnancy gingivitis

The dental professional should look for:

- Increased tendency for gums to bleed on gentle probing.
- Gingivae – blue-red, shiny, swollen, and smooth (due to increased vascular activity).
- Epulis formation (also known as *pregnancy tumour*) in severe cases, though rare.

An epulis (Figure 20.1) is a localised area of swollen interdental papilla, which may or may not contain pus. It can be found anywhere in the mouth, but is most commonly seen in the anterior regions. There may be more than one present and it is important to reassure the patient that there is no likelihood of malignancy. The OHE should ensure that the dentist has seen the epulis and be able to tell the patient that it will almost certainly disappear after birth. Very occasionally, an epulis persists and surgical removal is necessary at a later date.

Management of pregnancy gingivitis

The OHE should stress the importance of good oral health in toothbrushing, anti-plaque agents, and interdental cleaning, but should also advise that even with improved oral hygiene, pregnancy gingivitis sometimes persists until breastfeeding has finished and hormone levels have returned to normal. This becomes more significant if there is a progression to periodontal disease.

Remember! The primary causes of pregnancy gingivitis and epulis formation are the enzymes and toxins of mature plaque. Hormonal change is a secondary factor.

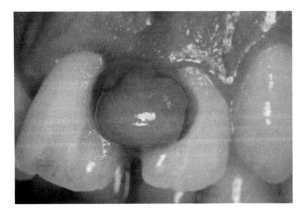

Figure 20.1 Pregnancy epulis. Source: Professor M.A.O. Lewis, Cardiff University. Reproduced with permission of Professor M.A.O. Lewis.

Periodontal infection

Research [4] shows that untreated periodontal infection (i.e. anaerobic bacterial infection in pockets) during pregnancy can result in adverse pregnancy outcomes such as:

- High blood pressure (pre-eclampsia).
- Premature birth.
- Low birth weight.

It is thought that these conditions occur because bacteria and their by-products can travel through the blood from the site of periodontal disease to the womb. However, there is still some debate about this and more research is needed.

Smoking-related conditions and diseases (see also Chapter 13)

The OHE should check whether a patient is smoking or vaping (or even chewing tobacco) and, if so, should advise and help her to stop. Advice and support should only be provided by dental staff that have completed a recognised cessation training programme. It is also worth contacting your local stop smoking service, which may also provide training and further information that can be given to patients [5].

In addition to the general negative effects of smoking on oral and general health, smoking during pregnancy also increases the risk of:

- Miscarriage.
- Stillbirth.
- Premature membrane rupture and birth.
- Ectopic pregnancy (fertilised egg implants itself outside of the womb).
- Placenta previa (placenta grows in the uterus and covers all/part of the opening to the cervix).
- Foetal growth restriction.
- Morning sickness.
- Infection.

Alcohol advice (see also Chapter 13)

As well as the adverse effects of alcohol misuse on general and oral health, there is a much greater risk associated with drinking during pregnancy. Alcohol passes through blood across the placenta to the growing baby. The baby cannot process alcohol as well as the pregnant woman, and too much exposure can seriously affect its development.

PREGNANT PATIENTS

Drinking during the first 3 months of pregnancy increases the risk of miscarriage, and drinking too much at any stage can cause foetal alcohol syndrome (FAS) leading to:

- Restricted growth.
- Facial abnormalities.
- Learning and behavioural disorders.

Pregnant patients should be advised that it is safer not to drink any alcohol if they are pregnant, or planning to become pregnant, because it can damage a growing baby [1].

SUMMARY OF ADVICE FOR PREGNANT WOMEN

The OHE should stress the following points to pregnant patients:

- Try to make time for oral care at a time of day when sickness is not present (sometimes a small-headed brush will help avoid nausea when brushing).
- Use a fluoride toothpaste (there is no known appreciable benefit to the developing baby in taking fluoride supplements, but fluoride paste will help prevent decay for the mother).
- Choose a softer toothbrush if gums are sore and bleeding, and use a *gentle scrub* or the *Bass technique* (see Chapter 19).
- Interdental care is even more important than usual. If bleeding is present, chlorhexidine mouthwash/gel may be used (see Chapters 14 and 19). Explain that this is not dangerous to the baby but should be used sparingly and for as short a time as possible to avoid staining and maternal anxiety. Although stains can be removed, many pregnant women are wary of ingesting chemicals in the gestation period.
- Keep up regular dental check-ups and hygienist visits.
- Never brush after vomiting, and rinse with water, fluoride mouthwash, or a solution containing sodium bicarbonate to neutralise the acid.
- Fluoride mouthwash may help combat the effects of nausea and frequent snacking.
- Stop smoking. Also, emphasise that once the baby is born, a smoke-free environment should be provided to avoid the effects of passive smoking (see Chapter 21).
- Avoid alcohol.

Remember! Partners also share responsibility for the mother's health, and that of the growing child.

REFERENCES

1. NHS (2019) *Start4life (Pregnancy)*. Available at: www.nhs.uk/start4life/pregnancy [accessed 2 September 2019].
2. NHS (2019) *Ready Steady Baby*. Available at: www.nhsinform.scot/ready-steady-baby [accessed 2 September 2019].
3. NHS Direct Wales (2017) *Your Antenatal Care*. Available at: www.nhsdirect.wales.nhs.uk/LiveWell/Pregnancy/ [accessed 2 September 2019].
4. European Federation of Periodontology (2013) *Gum disease, pregnancy and your baby*. Available at: www.bsperio.org.uk/publications/downloads/66_124600_pregnancygumdisease.pdf [accessed 2 September 2019].
5. Public Health England and Department of Health (2017) *Delivering better oral health: an evidence-based toolkit for prevention*. Available at: www.gov.uk/government/publications/delivering-better-oral-health-an-evidence-based-toolkit-for-prevention [accessed 30 April 2019].

PREGNANT PATIENTS

Chapter 21

Parents and guardians of pre-11 year olds

Learning outcomes

By the end of this chapter you should be able to:

1. Discuss teething and eruption dates with parents.
2. Advise on feeding, weaning, and diet.
3. Give advice on the ongoing care of deciduous and permanent teeth.
4. Advise on tooth-safe snacks and drinks for children.
5. Advise parents on the importance of regular dental visits.
6. Highlight the dangers of passive smoking.

INTRODUCTION

Parents and guardians will often ask for help on the care of their children's teeth, and parents of pre-11-year-old children is an important target group for the oral health educator (OHE) in which good habits can be established early on in life. (In this Chapter we refer to parents throughout, but the advice is applicable to any guardians of children.)

Visiting schools and clubs

As well as giving advice to individual patients, talking to children in schools or uniformed groups (e.g. Brownies, Cubs) often works well. Teachers will especially welcome dental talks as healthcare is included in the UK National Curriculum, and the OHE can build links with local schools to promote oral health.

Schools are also an excellent place to set up an exhibition or display (see Chapter 18), and the OHE could link together with other health professionals

Basic Guide to Oral Health Education and Promotion, Third Edition.
Alison Chapman and Simon H. Felton.
© 2021 John Wiley & Sons Ltd. Published 2021 by John Wiley & Sons Ltd.
Companion website: www.wiley.com/go/felton/oralhealth

in giving advice. Including parents can be even more beneficial in getting your messages across.

GENERAL ADVICE

Sugar-free medicines

Advise parents to buy/request sugar-free medicines from supermarkets, pharmacies, and GPs to help prevent caries (see Chapter 10).

'One hour before bed' rule

Encourage a 'one hour before bed' rule (i.e. no snacks or drinks 1 hour before bed). Toothpaste should be the last thing on the teeth before sleep. Only water should be provided if children require drinks through the night.

Passive smoking (see Chapter 13)

Passive smoking is especially dangerous for children and can increase the risk of:

- Childhood cancers, including leukaemia.
- Sudden infant death syndrome (SIDS), also known as cot death.
- *Otitis media* – middle ear infection, also known as *glue ear*.
- Poor lung function.
- Respiratory infections, such as asthma, bronchitis, and pneumonia.
- Mental retardation and behavioural, psychiatric, and cognitive problems.

SPECIFIC ADVICE TO PARENTS OF 0–3 YEAR OLDS

Parents of 0–3 year olds are often bombarded with advice from health professionals, as well as friends and family. However, much of this advice concerns the general wellbeing of the infant, and parents usually welcome specific information on the following topics.

Babies born with teeth

Natal teeth are teeth that are already present at birth, and are different from *neonatal teeth*, which appear during the first 30 days following birth.

Natal teeth are rare. They generally develop on the lower gum, where the central incisor teeth will appear, have little root structure, and are often wobbly and not well formed. They may cause irritation and injury to the infant's tongue when nursing and may be uncomfortable for a nursing mother. Natal teeth are often removed shortly after birth while the newborn is still in the hospital, especially if the teeth are loose and the child runs a risk of aspirating (*breathing in*) the tooth.

If natal teeth are not removed, the parent should be advised to keep them clean by gently wiping the gums and teeth with a clean, damp cloth. The baby's mouth should also be inspected frequently to make sure the teeth are not causing injury.

Eruption dates (see Chapter 1)

Parents should be advised that most teeth erupt from around the age of 6 months, but times are only approximate, and will vary from 4–12 months plus.

Teething

Some teeth grow with no pain or discomfort at all, but at other times the parent may notice any of the following symptoms:

- Sore, red gums where the tooth is coming through.
- A flushed cheek.
- Dribbling (and rashes from dribbling).
- Gnawing and chewing.
- Fretful behaviour.

You may have heard of other perceived symptoms, such as diarrhoea and fever. However, there has been no conclusive research to prove that these symptoms are linked to teething.

Advice on relieving teething pain

Each child responds differently to pain relief, and parents may find that they have to experiment with some of the following measures before finding what works for their baby [1]:

- Teething rings – to chew on. Can ease pain/provide a distraction. Some can be cooled in the fridge, but should not be put in the freezer (which can damage gums). A clean, wet flannel is an alternative to a teething ring.
- Chewing – chew healthy snacks, such as raw fruit and vegetables (e.g. carrot and apple), breadsticks, bread crusts and Bickiepegs® (which are sugar-free, vegan, and kosher). Parents should stay close by to avoid choking. Avoid rusks (and other foods that contain sugar).

- Painkilling medicine (paracetamol/ibuprofen) – for babies older than 3 months – to relieve pain/ temperature. Should be sugar-free and be specific to the age group. Aspirin should not be given to children under 16 years old.
- Comfort – comforting/playing with baby to distract them from pain.
- Preventing rashes – if baby is dribbling excessively, wiping their face and chin will help prevent rashes.
- Teething gels (sugar-free) – there is little evidence that teething gels are effective, and it is recommended that parents try non-medical options for teething first. If used, the gel must be specifically designed for young children. Gels contain a mild anaesthetic and are available from pharmacies.

If a parent thinks their child's behaviour is particularly unusual or symptoms are severe, they should be advised to consult their GP or call NHS 111 in England, Scotland and certain areas of Wales, and NHS Direct Wales (0845 46 47).

Effective cleaning of newly erupted teeth (see Chapter 11)

The application of a smear of fluoride toothpaste as soon as the teeth erupt is important in preventing decay.

Parents should be advised to clean gently around erupting teeth with a smear (the size of a grain of rice) of toothpaste (containing 1000 ppm fluoride) on a brush. And remember to advise spitting, but not rinsing.

Fluoride toothpaste (see Chapter 11)

No more than a smear of toothpaste (containing 1000 ppm of fluoride) should be used for children under 3 years old. Brushing with a fluoride paste, particularly at night, when the fluoride remains in the mouth, aids remineralisation, and is the most effective method of preventing caries in children.

Toothbrushing (see Chapter 19)

Some young children will refuse to cooperate with toothbrushing. Parents may mention that a previously cooperative baby takes delight in clamping their mouth shut at the approach of the toothbrush. Explain that this is a normal stage of development and is usually temporary.

The best approach is to ignore the rebellion and try to create diversions, such as new toothbrushes and brushing charts/competitions/games/rewards for older siblings. If there are no older children, parents can try brushing their own teeth in front of the little rebel (and making it look like fun!). Forcing the issue is rarely effective.

They should also be encouraged to spit out surplus paste, but not rinse.

Interdental cleaning (see Chapter 19)

As the teeth erupt and gaps close, interdental cleaning should be introduced. Flossing is the most appropriate technique at this age. Parents may find this hard to manage, so floss aids, such as handles, or floss picks may be more acceptable.

By introducing interdental cleaning in the early years it establishes this oral hygiene technique as a norm, something that is more difficult to achieve in adulthood.

Fluoride supplements (see Chapters 11 and 14)

It is the responsibility of the dentist to advise on this, and the OHE must follow that advice. Supplements are rarely advised unless the patient has a high risk of caries.

Comforters (dummies)

Comforters dipped in sweet substances should not be used.

Bottles and drinking cups

Only milk or water should be given in a bottle, and a baby/infant should not be left alone with liquid in a bottle.

Feeding from a bottle should be discouraged after a child is 1-year-old. This practice (apart from being unsafe) can result in the constant bathing of erupting tooth enamel in sugars. Prolonged use of a bottle and certain infant drinking cups (like feeder cups), which many parents favour because they do not leak when dropped, can result in early childhood caries, also known as *baby bottle caries*.

There is also concern about the affect feeder cups have on the developing muscles of the face and mouth.

OHEs could also recommend weaning babies on to a Doidy Cup (Figure 21.1), which has a slanted side to help the baby drink easily (see the liquid moving) and no lid, then move on to a normal cup.

Breastfeeding

Breastfeeding provides the best nutrition for babies until they are at least 1-year-old. However, breastfeeding does not work for all mothers, and those

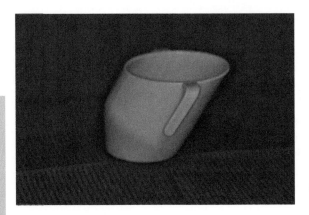

Figure 21.1 Doidy cup.
Source: Alison Chapman.

experiencing problems should be signposted to their health visitor or GP if they have not approached them already.

Breast milk substitutes

Formula breast milk substitutes should be discussed with health visitors, and if possible the OHE should obtain the latest advice and information from these professionals.

Note that soya milk and rice milk (sometimes recommended for allergy reasons) are high in sugar. Cartons with no added sugar can be bought for older children but they are not suitable for babies.

Formula milk should be given alongside solid foods until at least 1-year-old. Cow's milk, for drinking, should only be given after the baby is 1-year-old, and low fat milk is not suitable for children under two (fat is an important source of calories and important vitamins and minerals required at this age).

Weaning

The OHE should be able to provide general advice on weaning; particularly the role of sugars in the diet, and stress the importance of reading food labels (see Chapter 9), on specially formulated baby foods and drinks.

Small children (like much of the population) tend to graze, eating up to six times a day. Sugar-free grazing foods should be recommended, such as breadsticks, wholemeal toast, raw carrots, celery (to chew on), and plain yoghurt with mashed banana as a snack.

Parents should also be advised to suggest appropriate dietary advice to well-meaning family members and friends. Sweet treats should be avoided where possible and only given at pre-agreed times such as immediately after a meal/ once a week. Also, suggest that parents investigate snacks given at nursery and playschool before the child joins.

The OHE could also signpost the patient to their health visitor, GP and the NHS *Start4Life* website for more detailed advice on diet and weaning [2].

Visiting the dentist

The OHE should advise parents to take their children to the dentist as soon as possible so that they get used to the dental environment. The ideal time to begin dental visits is when the toddler's primary dentition is complete (at around 2–3 years). However, many infants are eager to show their teeth to the dentist at a much younger age, and this should be encouraged.

In the UK, there is no charge for NHS child dental treatment.

SPECIFIC ADVICE TO PARENTS OF CHILDREN AGED 4–6 YEARS

Children between 4–6 years old are still very dependent on parents for oral care and the OHE should be able to discuss with parents the following areas.

Eruption dates (see Chapter 1)

Explain that the first permanent molars (sixes) will erupt at the age of around 5–8 years, and stress the importance of cleaning. Patients are often unaware of these teeth erupting and think that no second teeth appear until a deciduous tooth has been lost.

Fluoride toothpaste (see Chapters 11 and 14)

Fluoride toothpaste should be used (1350–1500 ppm, pea-sized amount).

Toothbrushing (see Chapter 19)

Fones circular technique is very effective, but the parent must also be shown how to brush the lingual/palatal/occlusal surfaces. Explain that sometimes it is easier to sit with a child between the knees, their back towards the parent, tilting the head gently upwards. A child should not be allowed to run around or be left unattended with a toothbrush in its mouth.

Children should be encouraged to try brushing themselves, but the parent should brush the child's teeth as well. It could help to have a novelty brush for the child to use and a plainer brush for the parent to use. Children should be supervised when brushing.

Interdental cleaning (see Chapter 19)

Interdental cleaning should be taught as part of a daily oral hygiene regime. This is best done using floss on a holder or floss picks.

Fluoride supplements (see Chapters 11 and 14)

Fluoride supplements should be used (if appropriate). Fluoride mouthwashes are only suitable when the child is able to spit out, and many are not recommended for use by children under 6 years old.

Diet and sugar intake (see also Chapters 9 and 10)

It is important to establish good habits at this age, remembering that this age group is now mixing with peers and visiting other people's homes, where parents may not be responsible for meal planning and snacks.

Providing that a varied diet is being eaten, semi-skimmed milk can be drunk from 2 years old. Fully skimmed milk is not suitable until a child is 5 years old because it does not contain enough calories or vitamins.

Reiterate the importance of reading food labels and suggest that parents may be able to get together with friends in order to agree ground rules when giving food to each other's children. Plain milk or water should be advised in between meals.

SPECIFIC ADVICE TO PARENTS OF CHILDREN AGED 7–11 YEARS

Children in this age group are becoming more independent and like to brush their own teeth. It is generally thought that parents should supervise and help with cleaning until the age of at least 7 years [3]. Many parents, however, will think it is advisable to supervise all children of junior school age.

It is a good idea to involve both parents and children at this stage. Junior schoolchildren are particularly receptive to learning, and it is easy to capture their attention and involve them in selecting toothbrushes and thinking about their diet. A good range of resources and visual aids is essential (e.g. models showing the permanent teeth erupting).

Eruption dates (see Chapter 1)

Information on eruption dates is particularly important now as children lose more deciduous teeth, and permanent teeth are erupting.

Fluoride supplements (see Chapters 11 and 14)

Fluoride supplements should be used (if appropriate). Toothpaste should contain fluoride of 1400–1500 ppm (pea-sized amount), and the child should spit but not rinse. *At-risk* children between 10–16 years old can be recommended Colgate Duraphat® fluoride toothpaste (2800 ppm) on prescription twice daily. This needs to be discussed with the dentist before recommending and being prescribed.

Toothbrushing (see Chapter 19)

As the permanent teeth begin to erupt, the toothbrushing technique should be more defined, converting to the *short scrub* or *Bass* techniques, moving methodically around the mouth and making sure all surfaces are covered.

Power brushes are particularly effective in encouraging reluctant brushers, but still require supervision. The technique is less important than effective plaque removal. Not everyone likes (or can afford) these brushes, and you should explain that an ordinary brush could be used with equal effect. Be aware that battery powered toothbrushes may not have the desired brushing action.

As children take over their own oral hygiene and direct supervision declines, encouraging them to spend long enough cleaning can be a problem. Two-minute tooth timers can be employed, or perhaps listening to a favourite song, which lasts around two minutes. Some power brushes have timers which sound or vibrate every 30 seconds. This can be helpful to break the mouth into quarters to brush for two minutes in total. Occasionally, disclosing to check the child's effort can also be effective.

Interdental cleaning (see Chapter 19)

As the permanent teeth begin to erupt, interdental cleaning should be introduced if it has not been already. Floss, floss handles, or floss picks are most appropriate at this age although interdental brushes can be used if there is space. However, if there are wobbly teeth or gaps, an interspace brush can be employed in these areas.

Fluoride mouthwash (see Chapters 11 and 14)

Sodium fluoride mouthwash can be recommended for *at-risk* children between 6–10 years old (0.05% daily or 0.2% weekly).

Diet and sugar intake (see Chapters 9 and 10)

This age group is capable of understanding that sugar consumption causes tooth decay. They are receptive to alternative snacks and will enjoy taking part in games and competitions, which demonstrate how much hidden sugar is consumed. The UK National Curriculum encompasses education on health matters and many teachers will welcome a health professional who is prepared to present an exhibition on safer snacks for teeth (see Chapter 27).

Drinks become an increasingly important topic in this age group as the child will be capable of obtaining their own. Erosion should be explained, and the importance of avoiding frequent sipping of acidic beverages, such as fresh juice, squash, carbonated, and sports drinks.

Consumption of these drinks should be limited to mealtimes and without swishing around the mouth. Drinking through a (non-plastic) straw is recommended where practical and serving the drink chilled. Cold drinks tend to have a higher pH (i.e. more acidic) than warm drinks, and the straw places the liquid further to the back of the mouth.

Gum disease prevention

Parents are often focused on preventing caries and forget about gingival health. A surprising number of children in this age group present with gingivitis, and this becomes even more of a problem if an orthodontic appliance later becomes necessary.

Children of this age will enjoy using disclosing tablets or solution, but remember that this can be messy and permission for this should be obtained from parents. If you are visiting a school, check their policy on this type of intervention, especially if disclosing tablets are to be taken home.

REFERENCES

1. NHS choices (2019) *Tips for helping your teething baby*. Available at: www.nhs.uk/conditions/pregnancy-and-baby/teething-and-tooth-care/ [accessed 3 September 2019].
2. NHS (2019) *Start4life (Baby)*. Available at: www.nhs.uk/start4life/baby/ [accessed 2 September 2019].
3. Levine, R.S. & Stillman, C.R. (2009) *The Scientific Basis of Oral Health Education*, 6th edn. British Dental Journal, London.

Chapter 22

Adolescent and orthodontic patients

Learning outcomes

By the end of this chapter you should be able to:

1. Give specific oral health instruction to adolescent and orthodontic patients.
2. Advise and signpost on healthy snacks and drinks, smoking/alcohol/drugs.
3. Offer guidance on sports mouthguards.
4. Advise on the care of orthodontic appliances.
5. Explain *Angle's classification*.

ADOLESCENTS

Between 11 and 19 years old, young people begin to take more responsibility for their lives. Changing to secondary education is regarded as a milestone in the UK, and children begin to challenge parental control and involvement in their general wellbeing.

By the mid-teenage years, adolescents have a full adult dentition (except for third molars/wisdom teeth), and may present with the same problems as adults (e.g. gingivitis, caries, and erosion).

Young people in this target group will have opinions on what and when they eat, and peer pressure is strong. Media influence (especially social) can play a large part in determining what the latest trend will be. Adolescents also go through growth spurts during these years and are frequently hungry between meals, often resulting in unhealthy snacking.

Basic Guide to Oral Health Education and Promotion, Third Edition.
Alison Chapman and Simon H. Felton.
© 2021 John Wiley & Sons Ltd. Published 2021 by John Wiley & Sons Ltd.
Companion website: www.wiley.com/go/felton/oralhealth

Treating adolescents

When dealing with this age group the oral health educator (OHE) should remember the following points:

- It is best to tackle one problem at a time (e.g. gingivitis). Dealing with too many problems at once is impractical for the professional and could be too much for the patient to cope with.
- Target the young person rather than the parent (be tactful and remember that parents may wish to be involved or kept informed).
- Never patronise or talk down to teenagers. Treat them as adults and they will usually respond appropriately.
- Try to find acceptable methods of communication/motivation – it may be more difficult to motivate boys, particularly in their early teens. Try finding a topic that interests them and relate it to their dental health. As boys and girls become more interested in their health and appearance, they may become more motivated.
- Remember that peer groups have an important part to play at this age – talking to adolescents in school or uniformed groups often works well and teachers/leaders may welcome dental talks as healthcare is included in the UK National Curriculum. Advice can be associated with badge work in groups like Scouts and Guides.
- Intra-oral mouth piercing should be discouraged. Tongue bars and balls are known to damage teeth and cause recession (see Chapter 6). If already *in situ*, then oral health instruction will be required using a toothbrush or interspace brush to clean around them. Patients should be encouraged to either remove them or replace them with a plastic version to minimise damage.
- Be aware of bulimia and anorexia – look for signs (e.g. weight obsession, dramatic weight loss between appointments, and tooth erosion). Erosion in this situation is commonly seen on palatal and lingual surfaces, and the dentist may be the first health professional to identify a possible eating disorder. Careful and sensitive management is required.
- Be aware of smoking, alcohol, and drug misuse. This can be a very sensitive topic, and a source of friction between adults and parents (see Chapter 13).
- This age group tends not to be future-orientated, and so talk about what's happening to them now; bad breath, stained teeth, rotten teeth, pain, gums bleeding when eating etc.

Consent

In England, Wales and Northern Ireland, children under 16 can consent to their own treatment if they are believed to have sufficient intelligence, competence, and understanding to fully appreciate what's involved in their treatment (known as the *Gillick competence)*. Otherwise, someone with parental responsibility can consent for them [1].

If a competent child under 16 insists that their family should not be involved, their right to confidentiality must be respected, unless such an approach would put them at serious risk of harm.

Once children reach the age of 16–17 years, they are entitled to consent to their own treatment, as they are presumed to have sufficient capacity to decide on their own medical treatment. This can be overruled only in exceptional circumstances, where there is sufficient evidence to suggest otherwise, and then someone with parental responsibility can consent for them.

Advice for adolescents

Advice for adolescents should include the following topics [2].

Regular dental/orthodontic check-ups

Remember that until now most youngsters have attended the dentist regularly in family groups. When they leave home for university or take responsibility for their own lives, regular dental attendance may lapse. Therefore, stress the importance of:

- Regular check-ups (even if seeing orthodontist).
- OHE visits.

Effective cleaning (see also Chapters 14 and 19)

Advice on effective cleaning should include:

- Toothbrushing – teenagers can usually cope with the *Bass technique*, but be flexible and do not insist on a particular technique if the patient is cleaning effectively.
- Toothbrushes – many teenagers use power brushes. Be prepared to demonstrate the use of these, and advise on ordinary toothbrushes (size, texture, and frequency of renewal).
- Toothpaste – a fluoride paste (1400–1500 ppm) is important – check whether too much is being used. Be prepared to explain how it works and stress not to rinse after brushing. At-risk children over 16 years old can be recommended Colgate Duraphat® fluoride toothaste (5000 ppm) on prescription (twice daily).
- Interdental cleaning – explain why it is important (using the patient's own mouth to show swollen, bleeding gums, pictures, or commercial leaflets). Demonstrate using interdental brushes or floss.
- Mouthwashes – important if there is a high caries rate or an orthodontic appliance is being worn.
- Topical fluoride varnish – applied by the dentist/dental care professional. Be prepared to talk about this and how it can benefit the patient.

Dietary advice (see also Chapters 9 and 10)

Advice on diet should include:

- The importance of a balanced diet – healthy snacks and drinks, low in sugars.
- Chewing a sugar-free gum (containing xylitol) – after meals where possible (school policy on gum and wearing of orthodontic appliances must be taken into consideration).
- Snacks. Adolescents should be made aware of the potential harm to the oral cavity and general health of snack foods, including:
  - Chocolate, biscuits, and cakes.
  - Cereal, fruit, and nutrition bars – often high in sugar, though designed to appear healthy.
  - Crisps and savoury snacks – some are high in sugar, and labels should be studied.
  - Fizzy drinks – especially when sipped, as maintains contact with teeth over long periods.
  - Sports and energy drinks – many have high sugar content.
  - Diet drinks – although low in sugar or sugar-free, they still contain preservatives, such as citric and phosphoric acid, which can lead to erosion.
- These can also promote a craving for sweetness, which can lead to other health issues, such as obesity.

Anti-smoking/alcohol/drug advice (see Chapter 13)

Early teens is an excellent time to give anti-smoking guidance, as well as advice on alcohol and drugs.

Oral piercing advice

The OHE should advise on oral hygiene procedures if a patient has oral piercings or is considering them, and should provide the following advice:

- Use a reputable practitioner.
- Choose plastic versions, with flat backs/securers.
- Brush tongue, studs, and barbells twice daily with a soft toothbrush.
- Remove studs monthly, clean thoroughly and check regularly to make sure intact.
- Do not use ordinary jewellery cleaners (irritant properties).
- Take care when eating and do not fiddle or play with studs.
- If infection, swallowing or breathing difficulties occur, remove if possible, and seek urgent medical help.
- Visit the dentist if a tooth is chipped or damaged by a stud.

Sports mouthguards

Mouthguards are strongly advised for players of contact sports like rugby, hockey, martial arts, and lacrosse that involve high-impact physical contact.

By acting as shock absorbers, sports mouthguards can provide significant protection against injuries, which can occur directly from trauma or indirectly from tooth-to-tooth contact by cushioning and distributing forces that would otherwise result in serious dental injuries like bone fracture or even life-threatening situations. They also prevent damage to the oral soft tissues, which may occur from impaction against the teeth.

There are three main types of sports mouthguards that the OHE should be able to advise on: stock, mouth-formed, and custom-fit.

Stock mouthguards

The OHE should advise against these mouthguards. Stock mouthguards are inexpensive and available from most sports shops, but they are only available in limited sizes and do not fit very well. They also offer the least amount of protection as they are not made specifically to fit the grooves and contours of individual dentition. They cannot be adjusted and are likely to move around the mouth. If a guard does become dislodged, there is a chance it can block the airway.

Mouth-formed mouthguards

Mouth-formed mouthguards are also available through sports shops and are relatively inexpensive. They offer significantly more protection than stock guards, and are boiled to soften before moulding around a player's teeth and gums.

Custom-fit mouthguards

Custom-fit mouthguards are available through dental services and specialist companies, and offer the greatest protection (Figure 22.1). They provide a better fit than the other types, allow the player to breathe and speak more easily, and are more comfortable than mouth-formed mouthguards.

They are created in a dental laboratory from a patient's dental impression and involve two dental visits: one to get a dental impression and the second for fitting. If ordering through a specialist company (such as opro), the wearer is sent a home impression kit (according to the protection level and design chosen) to create a mould, which they send back to produce their mouthguard that is then posted back to the wearer.

They are the most expensive type of sports mouthguards, which can be a consideration if the patient's mouth is still changing. It is also possible to construct mouthguards for patients undergoing fixed orthodontics through the dentist.

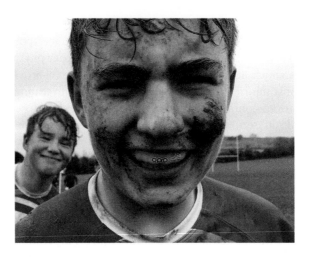

Figure 22.1 Custom-fit mouthguard. Source: Simon Felton.

THE ORTHODONTIC PATIENT

Orthodontics is the treatment of irregularities in the teeth and jaws, and the need for treatment is based on preventive, cosmetic, and functional considerations. As an OHE, you will not be expected to understand why orthodontic treatment is carried out and how it works, but some background information is useful.

Many adolescents have orthodontic appliances (Figure 22.2), and the OHE should be prepared to give advice on the care and cleaning of appliances and efficient mouth cleaning whilst the appliance is in place – including interdental cleaning and the use of fluoride mouthwash.

Deciding on orthodontic treatment

The orthodontist will take the following points into consideration when determining treatment:

- Skeletal pattern.
- Occlusion (i.e. how the upper and lower teeth meet). When assessing this, the true positions of the maxilla and mandible are taken into account. Measurements are taken to determine whether it is the jaws or the teeth in the alveoli that are misplaced. A lateral skull radiograph is taken to assist diagnosis. This shows the bones of the skull from the side, and the use of a filter allows the shadow of the soft tissues to be seen.
- Teeth. Two patterns (molar and incisal relationships) are considered. The position of the teeth is classified by *Angle's classification*.

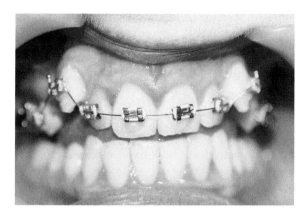

Figure 22.2 Mouth with orthodontic fixed appliances. Source: [3]. Reproduced with permission of Wiley-Blackwell.

Angle's classification

Angle's classification is used to describe the relationship of the molars in occlusion [4]. Dental nurse students using orthodontic patients as case studies may wish to go into this in more detail (see Chapter 27).

Angle's classification defines the extent of overbite and overjet:

- Overbite: the vertical overlap of the upper incisors over the lower incisors.
- Overjet: the horizontal distance between the upper anteriors and the lower anteriors.

Class I
Normal relationship where the lower 6 cusp tip bites half a cusp width in front of upper 6. The overjet and overbite are 2–4 mm.

Class II
The lower 6 is less than half a cusp tip width in front of the upper 6. Upper centrals are in front of lowers. This class has two divisions:

- Division 1 (also known as Class II, div 1). Upper teeth are much further forward than lowers, usually because of overcrowding. This tends to accentuate the upper teeth, the upper anteriors being *proclined* (protruding).
- Division 2 (also known as Class II, div 2). Overcrowding causes upper (and sometimes lower) incisors to retrocline (*lean back*) and sometimes the lowers also. Typically, the laterals overlap centrals and cause problems as there is nothing to restrain the lower anteriors that overerupt and bite into the palate, while upper incisors bite into the labial gingivae. Lower anteriors can have an *organ pipe* appearance.

Class III

Lower teeth are in front of the uppers, with the lower 6 more than half a cusp tip width forward. The bite is either edge to edge, or a reverse overbite. This can be due to oversized lower teeth, stunted maxillary growth or overgrowth of the mandible.

Advice for the orthodontic patient

Specific advice should be given for both fixed and removable appliances.

Fixed appliances

Adolescents usually adapt to wearing fixed appliances well, but they need advice on keeping the appliance and natural teeth clean to avoid gum problems. They should use a special orthodontic brush or a small-headed, medium/soft textured brush.

Some patients may do well with a power brush, particularly if using one already. Great care must be taken around brackets, bands, and wires. Help may be required with interdental brushes, and if there is suitable space, guidance on inserting them carefully. Interdental brushes can also be used to clean around the individual brackets, which can become plaque traps. Interspace brushes can be useful to clean around brackets or in the spaces created by extractions.

Also, promote the use of fluoride toothpaste. Advise that the use of a fluoride mouthwash can help avoid demineralisation around brackets and should be carried out at a different time to brushing.

As for diet, stress the usual dietary advice with reference to snacking, avoiding sugars wherever possible and difficult-to-eat foodstuffs (e.g. toffees, chewing gum). For drinks, the same advice applies as with adolescents, and also encourage the use of reusable straws.

Patients should attend regular orthodontic/dental check-ups, report discomfort promptly, and may be given dental wax to use on any wires that may otherwise traumatise the buccal mucosa. Should a bracket become loose, it is important that advice is sought from the orthodontist as soon as possible.

Retainers should be fitted after active treatment to prevent relapse (teeth moving back in original position). These should be worn as recommended by the orthodontist. Some patients will have fixed retainers usually behind the anterior teeth, which will need careful cleaning as they can become food traps and susceptible to calculus build-up. Interdental cleaning can be carried out using interdental brushes, or if these don't fit, then rubber toothpicks.

Removable appliances

Removable appliances should be worn at all times, except when cleaning the appliance or if advised otherwise by an orthodontist. When not being used they should be kept in water in a special orthodontic box.

Advise cleaning twice-daily at the same time as normal toothbrushing. The appliance should be held in the palm of the hand over a basin of water and brushed with soapy water using either a soft toothbrush or a soft nailbrush. Care should be taken to remove all food debris and plaque from around the wires/springs, before rinsing and replacing. The appliance can also be removed and rinsed after eating. Suggest weekly disclosing before removing the appliance to highlight problem areas (see Chapter 19).

Patients should also avoid very hard and sticky foods (e.g. toffees, chewing gum), and fizzy drinks and fruit juices should only be drunk at mealtimes.

Broken or lost appliances should be reported to the orthodontist straight away. An excellent standard of toothbrushing should be maintained, and stress the importance of gingival health whilst the appliance is being worn. Daily interdental cleaning should also be part of a good oral hygiene regime.

REFERENCES

1. NHS (2019) *Children and young people. Consent to Treatment.* Available at: www.nhs.uk/conditions/consent-to-treatment/children/ [accessed 4 September 2019].
2. Levine, R.S. & Stillman, C.R. (2009) *The Scientific Basis of Oral Health Education,* 6th edn. British Dental Journal, London.
3. Hollins, C. (2008) *Basic Guide to Dental Procedures.* Wiley-Blackwell, Oxford.
4. Ireland, R. (2004) *Advanced Dental Nursing.* Blackwell Science Ltd, Oxford.

Chapter 23

Older people

Learning outcomes

By the end of this chapter you should be able to:

1. Define who older people are and advise on the benefits of a healthy mouth to them.
2. Be aware of the dietary requirements of older people.
3. Recognise barriers to dental visits and how to break these barriers down.
4. State particular oral conditions of which the group is prone.
5. Advise patients and carers on overcoming problems, including advice on dentures.

WHO ARE OLDER PEOPLE?

A generation ago, nobody over 50 years old in the UK would have objected to being classified as old.

Things have changed dramatically over the last few decades. Diagnosis and treatment of many illnesses have vastly improved. People are living longer, eating more healthily, and are keen to improve or maintain their health. Today, many people over 70 years old would not consider themselves as old.

Until recently in dentistry, older people were associated with being edentulous (having no natural teeth), or partially dentate (having some natural teeth), although of course both can apply to people of any age. It is now increasingly common for dental professionals to treat patients in their 80s and 90s who have all their natural teeth.

Basic Guide to Oral Health Education and Promotion, Third Edition.
Alison Chapman and Simon H. Felton.
© 2021 John Wiley & Sons Ltd. Published 2021 by John Wiley & Sons Ltd.
Companion website: www.wiley.com/go/felton/oralhealth

British Dental Association classification of older people

The British Dental Association (BDA) describes older people as falling into three groups [1]:

1. *Entering old age*. Those who have completed careers in paid employment and/or child rearing. This is a socially constructed definition of old age, including people as young as 50 years old, or from retirement age. These people are active, functionally independent, and may remain so into late old age.
2. *Transitional phase*. Between a healthy, active life and frailty (functionally dependent). Often occurs in seventh or eighth decades, but can occur at any age.
3. *Frail older people*. Vulnerable as a result of:
   - Health problems (e.g. stroke, dementia).
   - Social care needs.

Of course, transition through these stages is relative, and one person may be active and independent at 85, whilst another may be frail at a much younger age.

UK adult dental surveys

In the UK, adult dental surveys take place approximately every 10 years. The following comparison between the last three UK adult dental surveys shows that dental treatment and its uptake by older people in the UK population have improved considerably:

- 1988 survey [2] – 80% of over 75 year olds had no natural teeth.
- 1998 survey [3] – 58% of over 75 year olds had no natural teeth.
- 2009 survey [4] – 30% of 75–84 year olds had no natural teeth (47% of adults over 85).

Benefits of a healthy mouth

The benefits of a healthy mouth in the older patient include:

- Allows enjoyable eating of regular, nutritious meals.
- Promotes confidence in appearance, eating, and speaking in public.
- Permits clear speech.
- Prevents oral infection that may affect general health – denture wearers are prone to denture stomatitis, angular cheilitis, and oral candidiasis (see Chapter 8).

OLDER PEOPLE

Diet and nutrition (see Chapter 9)

Healthy eating at any age is vital to good health and fitness. Older people generally have slightly lower energy requirements than younger adults, but still require a balanced diet, with greater emphasis on:

- Vitamin C (fruit and vegetables).
- Vitamin D (from sunlight or supplements).
- Calcium-rich foods to help avoid osteoporosis (low-fat dairy products).
- Carbohydrates (pasta, rice, and cereals).

Some older people have a greatly reduced appetite and should be encouraged to eat well, while others may be overweight which may restrict their mobility, and should be encouraged to lose weight. Some find that they can no longer eat large meals and tend to opt for small, frequent snacks, in which case healthy snacks should be promoted.

Barriers to a good diet

Changes in the following circumstances can result in a poor diet for the older person in particular:

- Death of a spouse.
- Reduction in physical activity/mobility (see Chapter 9).
- Failing health or eyesight.
- Illness.
- Xerostomia – drug- or age-related (see Chapter 7).
- Deterioration of smell or taste senses.
- Physical disability (unable to shop and go out).
- Poverty.
- Discomfort from ill-fitting dentures.
- Lack of awareness and information on oral health and nutrition.

Any of these circumstances may cause older people to skip regular, well-balanced meals and snack on easy-to-prepare (*ready meal*) alternatives, which are often high in sugar. Also, many older people grew up in an era when adding sugar to tea and coffee was the norm and find it difficult to break this habit.

Advising on sugar-free options (see Chapter 10)

By advising on sugar-free snack options, it may be possible to reduce the risk of caries by reducing their intake of free sugars in the following ways:

- Using sugar substitutes in cooking and drinks.
- Eating sugar-free sweets (some older people continually suck sweets to help dry mouths).
- Chewing sugar-free gum (if non-denture wearers).

OLDER PEOPLE

Fluoride (see Chapters 11 and 14)

Older people may benefit from the use of a fluoride mouthwash or toothpaste with higher fluoride content. Mention the availability of toothpaste prescriptions (containing 2800 or 5000 ppm of fluoride) – free for people over 60 years old in the UK.

Barriers to dental treatment

Some older people may find it difficult to attend dental practices that lack:

- Parking facilities.
- Ground floor surgeries.
- Wheelchair access.
- A bus route (to the practice)

Certain common medical conditions also cause mobility problems/difficulties in keeping appointments (see Chapter 24), including:

- Angina and other heart problems.
- Strokes.
- Parkinson's disease.
- Arthritis.
- Cancer.

Older patients who are carers may find it difficult to attend as they are not able to leave their own patient.

Breaking down the barriers

The OHE can help patients with poor mobility and physical impairment in the following ways:

- Suggest, or help arrange, domiciliary visits for those who are unable to attend a practice. However, bear in mind lone working protocol, medical emergencies and any consent issues. Try to form links with local doctors to encourage attendance.
- Check medical histories for any changes in health and consult the dentist as necessary.
- Write brief notes on advice (and products) given so that the patients can take this home with them.
- Suggest/help with adaptations to toothbrushes for patients with limited manual dexterity (e.g. handles can be enlarged for easy grip by the use of foam rubber, bicycle handlebar grips, rubber balls, or adding silicone impression material). Power toothbrushes may help and be easier to grip, but people with severe arthritis (see also Chapter 24) may find them difficult to switch on and too heavy.
- Demonstrate the use of one-handed interdental cleaning devices, i.e. interdental bottle brushes, wood sticks, floss picks, floss handles, and rubber tooth picks (see Chapter 19).

OLDER PEOPLE

- Allow extra time in the clinic (e.g. for getting in and out of the dental chair and the room). Think about the time of day in relation to the person being able to get up, dressed, on a bus, and in for an 8.30 am appointment. Many older people may not wish to have an appointment late in the day, especially in the dark winter months.
- Some patients may be dependent on family members or neighbours for transport or support and some may have others dependent on them, so always check out the needs of carers or family members and try to factor these in also.

Oral problems of older people

Certain oral problems are commonly experienced by older people and any person with dentures (see also Chapters 5–8).

These include:

- Xerostomia.
- Denture stomatitis.
- Angular cheilitis.
- Root caries – common in older people as recession exposes root surfaces not protected by enamel. (The critical pH that dentine demineralises is 6.0–6.5. Advise reduced sugar intake between meals; sugar-free medicines; thorough daily interdental cleaning; fluoride mouthwash; gels, and toothpastes.)
- Sensitivity – due to recession.
- Mouth cancer (see Chapter 8) – more common in older people often as a result of smoking/alcohol consumption. Look out for unusual red or white patches and ulcers (which do not heal). If an ulcer hasn't healed within 3 weeks then consult a dentist. Stress the importance of annual dental examinations, even in the edentulous, and smoking cessation (see Chapter 13).
- Oral soft tissues, particularly the mucosa, become more fragile with age, and may be more prone to trauma. Reduced saliva can result in thermal trauma from hot drinks.

OLDER PEOPLE

DENTURE CARE

As an OHE you may be asked to advise patients and carers on denture care. If you see the patient in the practice it can be useful to use a disclosing solution to show where there is plaque present and how to brush it off (Figure 23.1 a,b).

Many people with full or partial dentures suffer problems due to ineffective denture cleaning and too frequent soaking of dentures in bleach or well-known proprietary solutions. The Oral Health Foundation has a good, clear infographic on daily care (Figure 23.2).

(a)

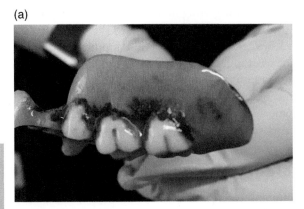

(b)

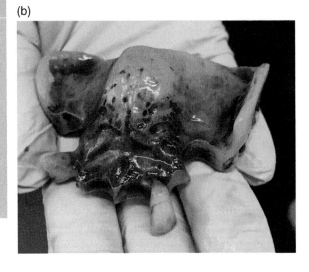

Figure 23.1 (a,b) Disclosed partial dentures. Source: Alison Chapman.

Older people in residential homes or those in poor health often have difficulty in keeping dentures clean. In residential homes, carers may be untrained or frequently changed, which can result in ineffective or inconsistent denture care.

Also, the OHE should look out for dentures that may not fit well, due to a loss of oral muscle tone, saliva or an impaired ability to chew or swallow (e.g. following a stroke), and should inform the dentist.

Advice to full denture wearers

Advice to older people and others who may be full denture wearers should include the following [6]:

- Daily mechanical cleaning of dentures – with a toothbrush (Figure 23.3), or denture brush and an effective, non-abrasive denture cleanser or liquid soap (not toothpaste).

Four simple steps to keep dentures at their best

1	**2**	**3**	**4**
BRUSH YOUR DENTURES DAILY	**SOAK YOUR DENTURES DAILY**	**LEAVE YOUR DENTURES OUT AT NIGHT**	**VISIT YOUR DENTAL PROFESSIONAL REGULARLY**
Use a non-abrasive cleaner, not toothpaste	Use a denture cleanser to remove more plaque and clean your dentures	Helps to relieve any soreness and prevent infection	Ensures your mouth remains healthy

A simple daily routine for clean dentures that promotes well-being and general health

Figure 23.2 Four simple steps to keep dentures at their best. Source: From [5]. Reproduced with permission of The Oral Health Foundation.

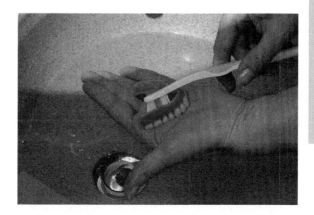

Figure 23.3 Denture cleaning. Source: Alison Chapman.

- Daily soaking in a denture-cleansing solution – to provide chemical breakdown of remaining plaque, plus disinfection.
- Do not keep dentures in the mouth overnight (except if there is a specific reason to do so) – especially important for frail patients, those at a higher risk of developing stomatitis, and those in care homes.
- Regular dental appointments.

Advice to partial denture wearers

Advice to partial denture wearers should be the same as with full denture care, with emphasis on:

- Removing dentures before cleaning natural teeth.
- Effective brushing/interdental cleaning of remaining teeth.

Advice to carers of patients with full or partial dentures

Carers for patients with full or partial dentures (including both family and professionals) should follow these steps when cleaning a denture or natural teeth:

1. Sit the patient comfortably in a back-supported chair, in good light. Stand behind or slightly to one side – be guided by patient's wishes. Have a mirror available.
2. Remove partial dentures (if natural teeth are to be cleaned).
3. Support the head, and gently draw back the lip. Use a small-headed or medium-headed toothbrush and appropriate toothpaste. Do not use too much toothpaste.
4. Brush only two or three teeth at a time – all surfaces, taking special care with any loose teeth. Any area that bleeds should be brushed more effectively.
5. Interdental cleaning is just as important as brushing and should be carried out at the same time. This may not be a realistic option, but should be encouraged.
6. If the patient tires easily, you may need to do one side of the mouth in the morning and the other side in the evening.
7. Finger guards are available from shops that sell aids for disabled people if there is a concern about being bitten.

OBTURATORS

OHEs may encounter patients who have had surgery for mouth cancer or have unrepaired cleft palates and wear obturators (specifically constructed appliances). These require specialist care, usually from the patient's oncology department or hospital dental department. They should be left out at night in water to prevent drying out, and cleaned using soap or denture cream, water, and a soft brush.

ADDITIONAL INFORMATION FOR CARE HOME MANAGERS

Care home managers should ensure that they have policies that detail plans and actions to promote and protect residents' oral health. They should be advised to follow NICE guideline [NG48] entitled *Oral health for adults in care homes*, which includes recommendations on [7]:

- Oral health assessment and mouth care plans (which should be undertaken on admission according to dental history).
- Care staff knowledge and skills.

OLDER PEOPLE

The care home should also have knowledge on the location and availability of:

- Local oral health and promotion services.
- Dental and community dental practices.

Care home staff should also:

- Consider issues of cross-infection – latex-free gloves should be worn.
- Make sure that patients have their own toothbrush (in good order), interdental aids, and toothpaste.
- Record any observed changes in the mouth or changes reported by the patient.

Smiling Matters: oral health care in care homes (CQC report)

The OHE, who has a particular interest in the oral health of care home residents, may also find interesting a report published by the CQC on the findings of 100 care home inspections after guidance was produced in 2016 by NICE. The document highlights the failings of many care homes to address the oral healthcare needs of the residents [8].

DEMENTIA

The OHE should be especially aware of the needs of patients who have dementia (including Alzheimer's disease), which affects memory and a patient's ability to communicate. It is important to establish a dental care programme at, or soon after, a patient has been diagnosed, and that patient agreement has been confirmed in writing by a person with capacity to make the decision. Consent must be given for every visit.

For patients with late stage dementia, consent should be obtained by the carer/family member who attends with them. The OHE should consult closely with their dentist, hygienist and practice manager about the treatment of such patients. Further advice and guidance can be found from the Faculty of General Dental Practice [9].

OTHER CONSIDERATIONS

Other considerations in the oral care of older people should include:

- Cost of treatment. This may worry the patient, and the OHE should be prepared to advise on:
  - Availability of free treatment.
  - Help with dental charges for those not on benefits.
  - Availability of good quality, reasonably priced, oral hygiene aids.

OLDER PEOPLE

- Visual/hearing impairment:
  - May be too proud to ask for help.
  - Unable to check own mouth after cleaning.
  - May not hear all instructions and advice.
- Difficulty with form filling. Be sensitive when offering help:
  - If you are completing the form ensure that you ask the patient the full question and record the full response.
  - When checking medical history, ask to see repeat prescription sheets and photocopy or scan these to include in their notes.

Remember! Older people were once as young and fit as you (may still be, or even more so). They should be treated with the same respect that you give to all patients and be offered the same treatment options.

REFERENCES

1. British Dental Association (2003) *Oral Healthcare for Older People: 2020 Vision*. British Dental Association, London.
2. Office of Population Censuses and Surveys (1991) *Adult Dental Health Survey (1988)*. HMSO, London.
3. Office for National Statistics (2000) *Adult Dental Health Survey (1998): Oral Health in the United Kingdom, 1998*. Stationery Office Books, London.
4. The Health and Social Care Information Centre (2011) *Oral Health and Function – A Report from the Adult Dental Health Survey 2009*. The Health and Social Care Information Centre, Leeds.
5. Oral Health Foundation (2018) *Four simple steps to keep dentures at their best*. Available at: www.dentalhealth.org/denturecareguidelines [accessed 22 January 2020].
6. Oral Health Foundation (2018) *White Paper on Optimal Care and Maintenance of Full Dentures for Oral and General Health*. Available at: www.dentalhealth.org/Handlers/Download.ashx?IDMF=81d96249-f307-4e21-aaea-1c861730710e [accessed 9 September 2019].
7. NICE (2016) *NICE guideline [NG48] Oral health for adults in care homes*. Available at: www.nice.org.uk/guidance/ng48/chapter/Recommendations#care-home-policies-on-oral-health-and-providing-residents-with-support-to-access-dental-services [accessed 9 September 2019].
8. Care Quality Commission (2019) *Smiling Matters: oral health care in care homes*. Available at: www.cqc.org.uk/publications/major-report/smiling-matters-oral-health-care-care-homes [accessed 5 February 2020].
9. Faculty of General Dental Practice (2017) *Dementia-Friendly Dentistry: Good Practice Guidelines*. Available at: www.fgdp.org.uk/dementia-oral-health-care-homes [accessed 19 December 2019].

Chapter 24

At-risk patients and people with special needs

Learning outcomes

By the end of this chapter you should be able to:

1. List patients at a higher risk than average of developing dental disease.
2. Explain circumstances associated with these patients that increase their risks of developing dental disease.
3. State how the oral health educator (OHE) can assist at-risk patients and people with special needs.

WHO ARE AT-RISK PATIENTS?

When talking about at-risk patients in the context of giving oral health education, we mean people who are at higher risk than the general population of developing dental disease, and/or find it difficult to manage oral health procedures.

Patients in this group include certain people covered in other target groups in this section, plus others who fit into the at-risk groups below:

- Medically compromised patients (those with chronic, systemic disease, and those on continual medication).
- People with physical or mental impairment.
- People of low socioeconomic status.
- Dental phobics, and those who never visit the dentist unless in pain.
- Severely compromised patients.
- People who smoke and/or misuse alcohol and other drugs.

Basic Guide to Oral Health Education and Promotion, Third Edition.
Alison Chapman and Simon H. Felton.
© 2021 John Wiley & Sons Ltd. Published 2021 by John Wiley & Sons Ltd.
Companion website: www.wiley.com/go/felton/oralhealth

Medically compromised patients (see also Chapter 8)

Medically compromised patients include people with systemic conditions that have oral implications, including:

- Lichen planus – a skin condition, which can affect the oral cavity.
- Diabetes (particularly periodontal disease).
- AIDS (including gingivitis, necrotizing ulcerative gingivitis, oral thrush).
- Epilepsy (the drug phenytoin can cause gingival overgrowth).
- Crohn's disease and colitis (gingivitis and ulceration).
- Sjögren's syndrome (xerostomia).

Many of these patients will be on continual medication, and may find it difficult to adhere to an oral health regimen. Some drugs may have side effects such as nausea and vomiting, which can cause dehydration and xerostomia in extreme cases (see Chapter 7).

Also, in some of these conditions, such as those with epilepsy and diabetes, the condition itself can cause problems in maintaining oral health or present difficulties in the surgery. In other conditions, treatment may be discouraged because of a risk from blood loss (e.g. patients with haemophilia and Von Willebrand disease).

Patients with diabetes

For patients with diabetes, observe the following guidelines:

- Keep to time with appointments, as the patient may have to eat at regular intervals to avoid hypoglycaemia (low blood sugar), which can be caused by too much insulin or skipping meals. Early signs to look for include shaking, dizziness or sweating, irritability/moodiness, anxiety, or nervousness.
- In rare, severe cases, hypoglycaemia can lead to a medical emergency, such as seizures, loss of consciousness, coma, and even death. The OHE should look for signs of confusion, drowsiness, and slurred speech.

Patients with epilepsy

Some patients with epilepsy have their condition well controlled by drug therapy, others less so. Taking phenytoin can lead to gingival overgrowth. Patients should speak to their specialist if this happens and ask to change their medication. The OHE should be aware of this side effect and be prepared to teach the patient how to place the toothbrush into the gingival margin to remove plaque. They should also consider teaching the patient how to use an interspace brush under the gingival overgrowth.

When a patient with epilepsy has a seizure, they can clamp their jaws together, biting their tongue causing ulcers and sores, and the OHE should also be aware that if the patient falls during a seizure they could damage their teeth. Some patients may require encouragement to keep regular dental/OHE appointments to help maintain excellent plaque control.

Epileptic seizures

Epileptic seizures can range from a temporary loss of awareness to loss of consciousness, body functions, and uncontrollable shaking/jerking. After a minute or two, the jerking movements should stop, and consciousness may slowly return.

In the event of a convulsive (*tonic-clonic*) seizure, follow these guidelines [1]:

- Protect the person from injury (remove harmful objects from nearby).
- Cushion the head.
- Look for an epilepsy ID card or identity jewellery, such as a wristband, which may say the patient has epilepsy and include information about seizures and medication.
- Aid breathing by gently placing them in the recovery position once the seizure has finished.
- Stay with the person until recovery is complete.
- Be calmly reassuring.

Do not:

- Put anything in the person's mouth.
- Try to move or restrain them unless they are in danger.
- Give them anything to eat or drink until they are fully recovered.
- Attempt to bring them round.

Call for an ambulance if any of the following apply:

- You know it is the person's first seizure.
- The seizure continues for more than 5 minutes.
- One seizure follows another without the person regaining consciousness between seizures.
- The person is injured during the seizure.
- You believe the person needs urgent medical attention.

Patients with haemophilia and Von Willebrand disease (VWD)

With modern treatments, these conditions (and other bleeding disorders) are usually well controlled, but unnecessary risks, which may lead to blood loss, need to be avoided. For example: dental procedures (i.e. injections) may put haemophiliacs at risk of haemorrhaging, and it is advisable to establish good oral health in childhood so that minimal dental intervention is necessary.

Patients with physical and mental impairment

These patients may require more time and patience as well as tact and special arrangements (where possible) when they attend for dental treatment. Some may need to be treated in special clinics or in their own homes by a community dental team. Those who can attend the surgery may need specially adapted oral hygiene aids or help to fill in forms.

The OHE must assess if an individual has the physical and cognitive ability to:

- Carry out effective personal oral care.
- Communicate needs to others.
- Access dental services.
- Make healthy, informed choices regarding diet.

Patients with physical impairment

Physical impairments include:

- Mobility difficulties (e.g. from birth, illness, an accident, obesity, pregnancy, or old age).
- Hearing impairment.
- Visual impairment.
- Limited manual dexterity (e.g. arthritis, cerebral palsy).
- Multiple sclerosis – variation in ability to clean depending on severity but may need a carer to clean.

Arthritis

There are more than one hundred different forms of arthritis and related diseases. The most common types include osteoarthritis (OA), rheumatoid arthritis (RA), psoriatic arthritis (PsA), fibromyalgia, and gout. All of them cause pain in different ways.

Arthritis can affect any of the joints in the body including the temporomandibular joint (TMJ), which connects the mandible to the skull. Arthritis in the TMJ can cause pain and difficulty when opening the mouth, and patients may have problems eating, talking, and undertaking basic oral hygiene procedures.

If the disease affects the hands, the patient can have problems holding and moving a toothbrush and cleaning interdentally. Manual toothbrushes, which have slim handles, can be adapted by using extra grip, such as tennis racket grip, tape to enlarge the handle, and to help with grip (see Chapter 19).

Powered toothbrushes can also help, as they tend to have wider handles and smaller heads. They can be used with the lips closed together, with little movement required. However, they may be too heavy for some.

For interdental cleaning, floss handles, picks and interdental brushes with longer handles may prove useful, including the TePe Angle™ and Curaprox Universal Holder.

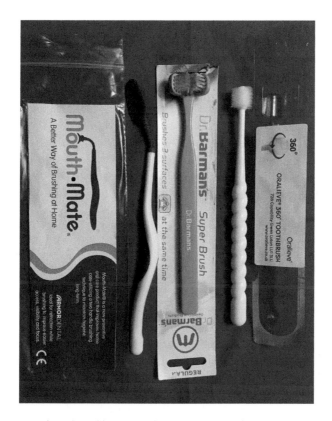

Figure 24.1 Special needs oral hygiene aids. Source: Alison Chapman.

For patients with limited dexterity, or where a carer needs to perform oral hygiene procedures, a three-headed DR Barman's Superbrush can be useful (Figure 24.1).

Patients with mental impairment

Patients with mental impairment include those with:

- Learning disabilities – for example, Down's syndrome, autism and associated disorders, head injuries, dementia (see also Chapter 23), and clinical depression.
- Inappropriate/challenging behaviour.
- Short attention span.

People of low socioeconomic status

OHEs working in deprived areas, hospitals, community dental services (CDSs), and dental access centres (DACs)/*walk-in centres* are more likely to help these patients (which include the homeless and recreational drug users), than those working in private practice.

Tact, understanding, and kindness are needed when helping homeless people. Remember that many patients have not always been in these circumstances. They often only request emergency treatment and will not attend again, thereby missing the opportunity for the OHE to provide further assistance. Homeless patients and those living in poverty may also find it impossible to afford oral hygiene aids, so it is a good idea to have free samples available to give out, where possible. Commercial companies may be able to help supply these, although if the patient is living on the streets they may have no facilities (such as running water and sinks) to carry out oral health procedures. A tactful, empathetic approach may be the key to persuading them to return for further treatment.

This group may also include people who misuse alcohol and take recreational drugs (see following text).

People who misuse alcohol and illegal drugs (see also Chapter 13)

The OHE should be particularly aware of patients showing signs of alcohol addiction and illegal drug and solvent use, and who could exhibit challenging behaviour as a result. You should have a basic knowledge of drugs (and substitutes used to treat addiction, e.g. methadone), and their effects on behaviour, oral and systemic health. You should also be able to offer brief interventions and signpost users towards further advice and support.

Certain OHEs may require special training (usually available for those working in the community), and must be prepared to adapt advice according to a patient's lifestyle and capabilities.

Patients with dental phobia

Patients with extreme phobia are also more likely to be encountered in a hospital or a community dentistry setting, since they would have been referred by dentists who do not have the resources to cope with their needs in the practice. The OHE must be guided by the instructions of the dentist, but can do much to help patients with phobias by using a gentle, understanding approach.

It is important to conduct oral hygiene sessions in a non-dental setting, free from dental noises and smells, and it may be appropriate for the OHE to not wear a uniform (which can be a barrier). Much time and patience is needed, and an empathetic questioning technique employed in order to ascertain the source and causes of their phobia. It may take a number of visits before the patient is comfortable enough to look at oral hygiene aids and discuss any treatment that may be required, but achieving a positive result can give the educator great job satisfaction.

Listen to their needs and work with them. Patients may not be able to look in a mirror at their own teeth and bleeding may cause great anxiety. Be prepared to adapt your normal instructions to make their visit as easy as possible, and with patience and regular appointments help them develop their trust in you.

Severely compromised patients

Generally, patients whose needs render them severely compromised live in specialised, residential homes, although some are able to live in their own homes with family members providing care along with social services.

These patients include those with:

- Paraplegia (from birth or accidents).
- Motor neurone disease.
- Dementia (late stages).
- Parkinson's disease (advanced).
- Multiple sclerosis (advanced).
- Palliative care needs.
- Debilitating strokes.

An OHE may be asked to give talks to carers about establishing and maintaining dental care for these patients (see Chapters 18 and 23). It is wise to find out exactly what is required before giving such a talk, to ascertain who the audience is, and what procedures are currently being adopted.

If you are required to give specific advice to individuals, the patient will need to be seen by a dentist and an oral health care plan established first. Home carers often have a difficult time and also need empathy, support, and advice.

Be prepared to advise on:

- Positioning the patient for effective and comfortable mouth care, including safety of patient and carer; standing behind the patient, gently tilting the head back and opening the lips with one hand, while cleaning with the other. A dental shield, mouth props, and tongue retractor (Figure 24.2) are available to help with this.
- Safe, effective plaque control (Chapter 19).
- Adaptation of oral hygiene aids.
- Preserving the dignity of the patient and encouraging them to do as much as possible for themselves.

Patients with heart valve defects

Historically, patients with heart valve defects who were prescribed antibiotics prior to treatment to prevent infective endocarditis were treated as medically compromised.

Currently, NICE Guidelines, reflected in British National Formulary (BNF) 55 (Section 5.1), now advise that antimicrobial prophylaxis (the use of antibiotics to

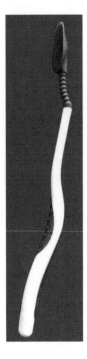

Figure 24.2 Tongue retractor. Source: Alison Chapman.

prevent infection) is no longer recommended for the prevention of endocarditis in patients undergoing dental and non-dental procedures [2].

Chlorhexidine mouthwash should also not be offered as prophylaxis against infective endocarditis to people at risk of infection undergoing dental procedures. Prophylaxis may expose patients to the adverse effects of antimicrobials when the evidence of benefit has not been proven.

Occasionally, a patient may present whose specialist insists on antibiotic cover, which should be respected and adhered to. The specialist should write a letter to the practice requesting this and it should be documented in the patient notes.

PHRASES USED FOR PATIENTS WITH SPECIAL NEEDS

Table 24.1 shows examples of acceptable and unacceptable phrases for certain patients with special needs.

Remember! All these patients require extra care, consideration, help, respect, and encouragement with oral health procedures. If the patient agrees, carers should be included, but your main point of focus should be the patient. Treat all patients as your equal (because they are).

Table 24.1 Examples of acceptable and unacceptable phrases for certain patients with special needs.

Acceptable phrases	Unacceptable phrases
Wheelchair user.	Wheelchair-bound.
Person with epilepsy.	Epileptic.
Person with disability or impairment.	Handicapped.
Hearing/speech impaired/impairment.	Deaf/dumb.
Visually impaired/visual impairment.	Blind.
Accessible toilet.	Disabled toilet.
Cerebral palsy.	Spastic.

REFERENCES

1. Epilepsy Action (2017) *First Aid for Seizures*. Available at: www.epilepsy.org.uk/info/firstaid [accessed 10 September 2019].
2. NICE Clinical Guideline 64 (2016) *Prophylaxis against infective endocarditis: antimicrobial prophylaxis against infective endocarditis in adults and children undergoing interventional procedures*. Available at www.nice.org.uk/guidance/cg64 [accessed 12 September 2019].

AT-RISK PATIENTS AND PEOPLE WITH SPECIAL NEEDS

Chapter 25

Minority cultural and ethnic populations in the United Kingdom

Learning outcomes

By the end of this chapter you should be able to:

1. Be aware of the population (in England and Wales) represented by minority ethnic groups.
2. List barriers in the uptake of dental treatment, and ways of breaking down these barriers.
3. List guidelines for producing suitable promotional material for this target group.

INTRODUCTION

Oral health educators (OHEs) will give oral health education to patients from minority ethnic groups, which is becoming an increasingly larger target group.

The 2011 Census for England and Wales recorded that 9.5% of the population was made up of black and minority ethnic groups compared to 7.85% in the 2001 census [1,2]. Older members of this population (particularly Caribbean) may have migrated here in the 1950s, but an increasingly large proportion is born in the United Kingdom.

It is therefore important to have some knowledge of the ideas and beliefs commonly encountered in people from these groups and to break down any barriers, such as language, that may exist.

Basic Guide to Oral Health Education and Promotion, Third Edition.
Alison Chapman and Simon H. Felton.
© 2021 John Wiley & Sons Ltd. Published 2021 by John Wiley & Sons Ltd.
Companion website: www.wiley.com/go/felton/oralhealth

BARRIERS TO DENTAL TREATMENT

Whilst it would be wrong to generalise, health and community personnel who work with minority ethnic groups are aware that the uptake of dental treatment in this section of the population is often below the national average.

There are a number of reasons for this, including:

- Older generations – may have never seen a dentist and may not see the need to take their children, or commonly only attend when they have a problem as they would in their country of birth.
- Bad experiences in country of origin – may have caused distress, and so reluctant to visit the dentist.
- Conflicting views in the family – concerning the importance of oral health.
- Lack of awareness of services and facilities.
- Communication/language barrier.

Breaking down the barriers

The OHE has a unique opportunity to break down some of these barriers in the following ways.

Meet with community leaders

Get to know local community leaders and religious figures, forge links and establish what help is needed and what initiatives could be taken to encourage regular dental attendance. Consider giving talks at local community venues (see Chapter 18), which can be tremendously rewarding.

Contact other professionals

Contact doctors, health visitors, practice nurses, and teachers who may already be involved with a health programme in the area. Oral health is a part of general health and it may be possible to join forces with other health professionals in giving advice on general health, such as:

- Diet/nutrition.
- Diabetes/heart disease.
- Betel nut chewing.
- Suitable oral health products.

Diet/nutrition (see Chapter 9)

Advice is often welcomed, but consult health visitors/school teachers first as there are differences in what certain religions/beliefs can and cannot eat. For example, the Muslim faith forbids the eating of pig and carnivorous animals. OHEs will also need to be aware of the timing of religious festivals that involve fasting, such as *Diwali* (Hindu) and *Ramadan* (Muslim).

Heavily spiced foods can contribute to tooth staining and there may be issues with abrasion. Find out what is in snack/drink items that are being consumed. Remember that lacto-vegetarian or vegan regimes may be adhered to by any nationality.

Diabetes and heart disease (see Chapter 8)

The OHE should be aware that diabetes is relatively high in Black Caribbean men and women (10% and 8%, respectively) compared with the general population (4% and 3%, respectively), which may have ramifications on oral and general health [3].

Heart attacks and angina are also more common in Asian people, and nearly a third of Pakistani men (31%) have angina compared with 13% of men in the general population. High prevalence of angina is also found in Indian women (15%), compared with the general population (9%). The prevalence of heart attacks is high in both Pakistani men (19%) and women (7%); in the general population, the equivalent rates are 10% and 5%, respectively [3].

Betel nut (paan) chewing (see Chapter 13)

Betel nut (and paan) chewing is a habit in certain cultures (particularly in Southeast Asia), and produces a red stain. It is used to relieve stress and is a mild stimulant (similar to tobacco smoking). Users should be given similar advice to smoking cessation and be signposted to their local NHS Stop Smoking Services.

Suitable oral health products

Think about what oral health products you recommend. Some may not be suitable for use by certain cultures. For example, certain saliva substitutes contain porcine (pig mucin), which is forbidden in Islam and Judaism, and certain mouthwashes contain alcohol, which is prohibited in Islam.

Language custom/how to address people

While it may be unlikely that you will learn languages to treat different patients, a little goes a long way in breaking down language barriers. For example, you could find out how to address, greet, and say goodbye to people in their native language and say *please* and *thank you*.

By making an effort, the OHE will have breached an important social/language barrier, broken the ice, and earned greater respect from the patient, who may now be more open to advice.

Produce suitable promotional material

Imagine if you were overseas, needed dental treatment, and were faced with a brochure about services that was written in Arabic?

When producing resources, bear in mind that each minority group has its own culture, traditions, and customs. It is possible to find dental leaflets translated into a number of different languages.

The OHE should also bear in mind the following points when producing material:

- Individuals in an illustration – should reflect all population groups.
- Written material should have the appropriate language. For example, Punjabi can be written using two different alphabets, depending on the country of origin.
- Pictures of foodstuffs – should relate to the culture and include suitable foods/labels.
- Pictures of people eating – must reflect the fact that some religions, such as Islam, would regard it as offensive to eat with the left hand.
- Certain symbols and icons are not universally recognised. For example, some cultures reverse the meaning of a tick or a cross on a questionnaire.
- Some cultures read from *right to left* or use picture language.
- Pilot material you have produced with a community leader before distribution.

MINORITY CULTURAL AND ETHNIC POPULATIONS IN THE UNITED KINGDOM

REFERENCES

1. Office for National Statistics (2013) *2011 UK Census of Population*. The Stationery Office, London.
2. Office for National Statistics (2003) *2001 UK Census of Population*. The Stationery Office, London.
3. Office for National Statistics (2006) *Health Survey for England - 2004: Health of ethnic minorities*. The Stationery Office, London.

Chapter 26

Other health professionals

LEARNING OUTCOMES

By the end of this chapter you should be able to:

1. List other health professionals who may be giving oral health advice to the public.
2. Confidently pass on your knowledge of oral health to these professionals who may be patients themselves, or who may be passing on advice to their own patients.

INTRODUCTION

The oral health educator (OHE) should be aware of other health professionals who give advice that can affect the oral cavity as well as the general health of patients.

It is very important that all providers give the same messages on both oral and general health matters to avoid confusion and conflicting advice among recipients, particularly regarding advice on diet and the effect of food and drink on the oral cavity.

From time to time the OHE may also be required to educate other health professionals and should feel confident in their own ability to do so.

WHO ELSE PROVIDES ORAL HEALTH EDUCATION?

Health professionals in a number of different sectors give oral health advice to the public. These professionals include:

- Health visitors.
- Community and hospital midwives.

Basic Guide to Oral Health Education and Promotion, Third Edition.
Alison Chapman and Simon H. Felton.
© 2021 John Wiley & Sons Ltd. Published 2021 by John Wiley & Sons Ltd.
Companion website: www.wiley.com/go/felton/oralhealth

- Social workers.
- Community/school nurses.
- Doctors and practice nurses.
- Hospital nursing teams.
- Rehabilitation teams – multidisciplinary teams (MDTs), which can include physiotherapists, occupational therapists, and speech and language therapists.
- Professional carers.
- Dieticians.
- Pharmacists.
- Teachers.
- Nursery leaders.
- Commercial organisations (companies selling oral health aids, etc.).
- Health journalists.

TEAM UP WITH OTHER PROFESSIONALS

The OHE should be aware of regular health events that they can get involved with alongside other health professionals (see also Chapter 32), such as:

- *Alcohol Awareness Week* – a week in November, run by Alcohol Change UK.
- *Mouth Cancer Action Month* – each November, run by the Oral Health Foundation.
- *National Smile Month* – each May, run by the Oral Health Foundation.
- *Stoptober* – each October, run by Public Health England.
- *World No Tobacco Day* – 31st May each year, run by The World Health Organization.

Such national and global initiatives often have local events, as well as there being other local government and community initiatives not linked to wider events. These are great opportunities to deliver information to a community, and for the OHE to become involved with other professionals who provide general and oral health education. For example, by setting up a display or an exhibition (see Chapter 27) within a general theme, such as a cancer, or by giving a talk to an important target group, including oral health professionals (see Chapter 18).

There is a lot to be learnt by listening to other health professionals in both their subject matter and in the way they deliver information, but the OHE should also not underestimate their own knowledge and experience, which can be passed on to other professionals.

The OHE should be aware of how professionals obtain information to pass on to patients and, in turn, may be able to help other professionals in sourcing information, learning aids, and even free samples. For example, some companies produce project material for use with schoolchildren, and it is worth asking dental representatives if anything like this is available for teachers. Information may also be sourced from leaflets in hospitals and health centres.

GIVING ADVICE TO INDIVIDUAL HEALTH EDUCATION PROFESSIONALS

Most patients, who are also health professionals, will see the OHE in a role of someone the dentist has suggested can help them, but other health professionals could see it as insulting that the dentist feels that their oral hygiene could be improved. A good initial approach with such patients can be to ask how they feel about their current oral hygiene habits and whether they feel change could be beneficial.

Careful lesson planning is vital, and should take into account the patient's profession (see Chapter 16). For example, if the patient is a dental professional, OHEs know that they can use dental terms. But if, for example, the patient is a dietician who will not necessarily understand technical dental jargon, the OHE should plan the lesson accordingly, perhaps asking the subject's opinion regarding dietary advice for patients.

It is assumed that because a patient is well educated and working in a health-related field, that they will be aware of the importance of oral health measures, such as interdental cleaning. However, this is not always the case, and sometimes considerable tact is necessary in finding out what dental aids/practices patients use/employ, and in persuading them that change could be helpful. An appropriate evaluation of each session should also be undertaken (see Chapter 16).

Having mastered the art of dealing with other health professionals, OHEs will find themselves less nervous in giving advice to the general public, and usually find that the same respectful, yet confident approach works well with everyone, even children!

OTHER HEALTH PROFESSIONALS

Chapter 27

Planning education case studies, exhibitions, and record of competence

Learning outcomes

By the end of this chapter you should be able to:

1. Acquire confidence to plan and carry out case studies.
2. Record the outcome of case studies (*record of competence*).
3. Have the knowledge to set up an exhibition or display (in conjunction with chapter 18).

INTRODUCTION

Oral health education students studying for a UK qualification are required to carry out (and record) case studies on patients who fall within the target groups covered in this section, or on patients for whom there is a specific concern about their oral health that needs addressing. Case studies are also a good method of establishing sound oral health education practices for all patient sessions (see Chapter 16).

Details of each session should be recorded using practical competence assessment sheets (PCAs), and patient records should include aims, objectives, and an evaluation of the outcome(s), which can be used as reflective practice to improve further sessions with patients and identify areas the oral health educator (OHE) needs to research for self-development.

Choosing oral health subjects

Carrying out oral health education requires much thought, input and dedication. Appointments can be quite personal, and can help the OHE get to know

Basic Guide to Oral Health Education and Promotion, Third Edition.
Alison Chapman and Simon H. Felton.
© 2021 John Wiley & Sons Ltd. Published 2021 by John Wiley & Sons Ltd.
Companion website: www.wiley.com/go/felton/oralhealth

patients well. In doing so, you can become an important catalyst in changing patients' oral health regimes.

Try to find patients who require a fair amount of help and encouragement (and who are likely to keep appointments). Discuss suitable patients with your dentist, hygienist, or supervising witness.

Patients will need to have either:

1. A number of things to achieve in order to improve oral hygiene, or
2. A special reason for improving oral hygiene.

Plan ahead

After selecting your patient(s), the next step is to arrange several appointments in advance, making sure that you have allowed around 30 minutes for an adult patient. For children, you may need slightly more or less time depending upon the age of the child and the problems to be tackled. Remember that children (particularly pre-school age) have a short attention span.

It is a good idea to ask for sufficient notice from your dentist before seeing a patient, in order to study their dental records and plan the session effectively. Having studied the patient's records and found what is required, guidelines on planning a session should be followed and a lesson plan written (see Chapter 16).

Putting yourself and the patient at ease (see also Chapter 15)

It is normal to feel nervous and apprehensive when talking to a patient, particularly if somebody else in the workplace is observing. However, once you have talked to the person, found out a little about them and planned what steps are required, the second visit (or patient) will not be nearly as intimidating. Remember that the patient may be more nervous than you.

Always greet patients warmly, introducing yourself with a smile, and invite them to remove outdoor clothing and take a seat (preferably in a comfortable chair in a setting free from dental equipment, noises and smells). However, this is not always possible – most hygienists and therapists carry out their sessions along with their clinical work, often with the patient in the dental chair. It is the educator's attitude, body language, and knowledge that put the patient at ease and helps achieve the desired results.

Do not expect miracles

Do not expect an instant change of attitude or behaviour in patients. It sometimes takes a few visits to get to know them and what goes on in their lives, before they are persuaded to change their behaviour. Therefore, be meticulous in obtaining as much background information as you can, which can be used in the opening greeting.

For example:

Hello, Mrs Jones, we have met several times when Mr Smith has been treating your children. My name is Ann, and Mr Smith has asked me to discuss little Freddy's diet with you as he has already had two fillings. By the way, how is Freddy enjoying his new playgroup? I remember you telling Mr Smith that he was apprehensive about starting there.

In that way, you have begun a relationship with Mrs. Jones, impressed her by remembering her conversation with the dentist, and given her a chance to chat about something other than Freddy's diet (may be relevant to his caries record), which will help to put her at ease. It is a good idea to keep a notebook with you and jot down points like Freddy's playgroup, but not anything you perceive as confidential between patient and dentist (and remember that the patient has every right to look at what you have written).

You will soon find that talking to patients is much easier than you imagined and probably one of the most rewarding aspects of the OHE's job.

Dealing with difficult patients

There will always be difficult patients who will grumble about everything and some who are even openly hostile. Often, aggressive behaviour is a cover-up for anxiety or fear (see Chapter 15). If you tell yourself that aggressive behaviour is concealing something in the patient's life that you do not know about and treat them with extra kindness and patience, more often than not they will respond positively.

Some teenagers can be particularly challenging – often they will avoid eye contact and it is difficult to establish a relationship with somebody who behaves in this way (see Chapter 22). Once again, tact and patience may achieve results, and seeing the teenager without a parent can help. You can always ask the patient's permission to include mum or dad at the end of the session to briefly explain the points you have made.

It may also help if you can find some common ground upon which to approach the teenager. For example, '*Have you noticed* (name of sporting hero's) *stunning smile? Wouldn't it be gross to see red, swollen gums and black teeth when (s)he is interviewed on TV?*' You could even have posters of sports or other personalities in the PDU, showing their beautifully cared-for teeth.

Patient records

After each session, you will need to record how the session went using a form provided by your qualification provider or devised by yourself (if you are recording sessions outside of a qualification).

Each record must be signed by a *supervising witness* who should be aware (through prior discussion) of your proposal, and has already approved your lesson plan.

Case study examples

Here are two examples of case studies undertaken by OHE students.

The patient with a number of things to improve

A 47-year-old patient had extensive complex restorations, in other words, large fillings, crowns, and bridges. Despite trying hard to improve her standard of oral health, she could not achieve effective plaque control; consequently, her gingival condition was poor and deteriorating.

One student saw her about six times, got to know her lifestyle and fired her with enthusiasm to improve her oral health. Under this guidance, the patient learned to use interdental brushes and Oral-B® SuperFloss™ effectively. She was also able to perform efficient plaque removal from heavily filled teeth using a power brush.

Both the OHE and the patient gained a great deal of satisfaction from the exercise, and the examiners liked the way she had tackled and explained her case study.

The patient with a special reason for improving oral health

Another student had a 15-year-old relative who was a patient at her practice, and who came into the category of *special care*. He had moderate learning difficulties and in her words: '*was about 9–11 years old in understanding and capability, but keen to improve*'.

The OHE, acting upon her dentist's instructions, decided that she would try to improve:

1. His toothbrushing – which left much to be desired, resulting in poor gingival condition.
2. His diet. He consumed numerous high-sugar snacks and drinks between meals, resulting in a high caries rate.

The OHE tackled both these aspects, which in ordinary circumstances would probably have been too much. It is often better to tackle one aspect of oral health at a time.

However, in this case, she had frequent access to the patient who cooperated and enjoyed the sessions. The OHE made large mouth models to demonstrate effective toothbrushing and helped him perform brushing techniques in front of a mirror. She also showed him how to use disclosing tablets and encouraged him with *before* and *after* photographs of his mouth.

When his brushing had improved, she taught him how to look at the labels on his snacks. When the time came to submit her case study, she was still working with him, and recognised how much more time was needed. However, she had learned a great deal about working with such a patient and was able to explain this in her write-up.

Exhibition or display (see also Chapter 18)

As part of your qualification, you will also need to carry out an exhibition or display in the workplace or outside in locations such as residential homes, schools, hospitals, clinics, and church halls. The exhibition or display must be self-explanatory, in case you are not expected to be there all of the time to answer questions.

There now follows some guidance notes on choosing a topic for your course qualification exhibition or display.

Choosing a topic

Try to choose a topic that is relevant to the practice or workplace.

Reasons for a choice of topic may be that either:

1. Your dentist or hygienist has noticed an aspect of patients' oral health that requires improvement. This can be targeted in your practice. For example, perhaps your dentist has strong feelings that all patients should floss regularly, but they or the hygienist has noticed that responses to their suggestions have not been good.
2. The practice could specialise in implants or orthodontics and a display on the maintenance of these could be very useful.
3. You are asked by friends who are teachers or health professionals to improve oral health knowledge in their class or with their patients. This is usually done outside of the workplace.

Examples of exhibitions/displays

Here are several examples of exhibitions/displays by former students:

1. In response to a request from a teacher who was a patient at her practice, an OHE set up an exhibition on *Tooth-friendly Packed Lunches* in a local primary school. The children came into an area, one class at a time in their lunch hour and the OHE stayed with her exhibition and answered questions from children and staff.
2. A student, whose teenagers were in a swimming club, noticed that young swimmers, many of whom were patients at her practice, continually sipped sports drinks whilst waiting for races. Her dentist had noticed a surprising rise in teenage erosion, and so she set up an exhibition on the subject and

took it to the local secondary school, before moving to the local swimming club premises.

3. A student found that when her grandmother went to live in a care home, the care workers did not seem to give oral hygiene much attention when helping her grandmother with her personal hygiene. She approached the care home and asked if they would be interested in her offering advice. She produced an exhibition about oral care for the carers, including how to clean dentures.

The possibilities are endless, but it is a good idea to pick a topic on which you and your dentist agree, and in which you have a particular interest. If you are interested in your topic, your enthusiasm will carry you along.

Exhibition plan (also see Chapter 18)

Having decided upon the subject of your exhibition, you need to make a campaign plan, enlisting the help of colleagues, if possible. For example:

1. What are my aims and objectives?
2. Who is the target group?
3. Venue – where shall I set it up?
4. When would be a good time to do it?
5. What resources should I use?
6. How should I evaluate its outcome? For example, following my exhibition:
   - 25 patients demonstrated that they could use dental floss effectively.
   - 20 patients said that they would try to use floss regularly.
   - Four patients would try to use another interdental method.
   - One patient would not change their behaviour.

REFERENCE

1. Levine, R.S. & Stillman, C.R. (2009) *The Scientific Basis of Oral Health Education*, 6th edn. British Dental Journal, London.

PLANNING EDUCATION CASE STUDIES, EXHIBITIONS, AND RECORD OF COMPETENCE

Section 6

Oral Health and Society

INTRODUCTION

This section looks at how society and behaviour influence the oral health of the nation.

It examines the issues of socialisation (particularly the impact that family and other social groups and institutions have on the oral health of individuals), and epidemiology – the study of the prevalence and distribution of disease within a population. It also looks at how evidence-based prevention (advice based on research studies) is driving oral health policy and practice.

Quality control in UK dental services is addressed, and the ways in which dental treatment can currently be obtained. It also examines similarities and differences between oral health promotion and education, and how promotion can help improve the oral health of the population.

The section concludes with a chapter on how to read and analyse research papers for students and professionals who want to keep up-to-date with the latest research findings and thinking.

Chapter 28

Sociology

Learning outcomes

By the end of this chapter you should be able to:

1. Define *sociology* and *socialisation*, and explain factors that influence the uptake of health care.
2. Define and differentiate between *primary* and *secondary* socialisation.
3. Explain what is meant by *values* and *norms*.
4. Show awareness of the UK Office for National Statistics' *Register of Social Groups* and give examples of social class differences within the population.
5. Explain what is meant by the terms *iceberg effect*, *victim blaming* and the *performance gap*.

SOCIOLOGY

Sociology can be defined as *the study of the structure and functioning of human society*.

In order to understand the uptake of dental treatment by the population of the UK, the oral health educator (OHE) needs to study the way that society functions and is structured.

Sociologists tell us that individual behaviour in the uptake of healthcare is influenced by:

1. Political and economic decisions and influences. For example, UK government funding changes to NHS Dentistry in 1990 resulted in many dentists entering the private sector. Consequently, many people marginally above the social benefits line could no longer afford to visit the dentist. This effect is still seen today.

Basic Guide to Oral Health Education and Promotion, Third Edition.
Alison Chapman and Simon H. Felton.
© 2021 John Wiley & Sons Ltd. Published 2021 by John Wiley & Sons Ltd.
Companion website: www.wiley.com/go/felton/oralhealth

2. Cultural influences. For example, refugees claiming asylum may not have been brought up to attend the dentist, or had a dentist available in their country of origin, and so do not go.

Socialisation

Socialisation is the process by which infants and young children become aware of society and their relationships with others [1]. From the moment of birth an infant begins the learning process. For example, in these early days, parents talk to babies, smile at them and very soon the baby responds and imitates smiles and sounds. So begins the process of socialisation.

The OHE needs to understand the two main stages of socialisation:

1. Primary socialisation – describes learning that takes place before starting school, beginning as soon as the child is born. Many sociologists think that beliefs and attitudes learned in these years are almost impossible to change in later life. This is when a child is very receptive to learning about topics such as toothbrushing and a healthy diet, and family life and behaviour. The child learns from:
   – Parents.
   – Close family members (grandparents and siblings) – about how to behave within the family. This learning is vital to establish healthy behaviour patterns. Children deprived of these early learning opportunities often grow up with behavioural problems.
   – The reconstituted family – many families are involved in relationship breakdown and repair, which can have a profound effect upon primary socialisation, with a child's learning being interrupted or changed.
   – Close friends and their children.
2. Secondary socialisation – refers to learning that takes place outside of the close family. This usually begins when the child starts nursery, preschool, or primary school, and is influenced by the ideas and practices of:
   – Teachers.
   – Peers.
   – Media.
   – Carers.
   – Healthcare professionals (including the dental team).

Within socialisation, *formal socialisation* is a term used to describe that which occurs in settings intentionally designed for socialisation, such as school, while the term *informal socialisation* involves assimilating the attitudes, values, and behaviour acquired in one's personal life from family, friends, and so on.

During educational years, the child should hopefully learn to behave acceptably outside of the home, according to the *values* and *norms* of society.

Values

The values of society are also referred to as collected beliefs (e.g. *society demands equality in healthcare for all individuals*). These are *ideals,* and the OHE soon becomes aware that in many aspects of dental treatment, as in life, there is no equality.

Norms

Norms describe the most common patterns of behaviour, but not everyone conforms to these patterns and they can vary according to country, culture, and ethnicity, for example. It could be said that it is the norm for people to brush their teeth twice daily or the norm to have regular 6-monthly dental check-ups in the UK, but this can vary depending on social status and background

Social classes

In UK society, there is still a social divide between the classes, which dates back to Victorian times when there were upper classes (employers and gentry) and lower classes (those who worked for them). In modern UK society, a person can still be classified according to their socio-economic status.

Table 28.1 shows the UK National Statistics Socio-economic Classification (NS-SEC) of analytical classes [2]. These social classes are not simple to analyse, and are designed principally for the purpose of epidemiological surveys (see Chapter 29). Surveys [3, 4] reveal that social class reflects values, norms, and beliefs held by different community groups, and these social factors influence behaviour.

For example, epidemiological studies and surveys have shown that people from higher social classes are generally, though not always, the most future-oriented (i.e. more likely to take preventive action, like visiting the dentist more frequently).

Table 28.1 National Statistics Socio-economic Classification (NS-SEC) of analytical classes.

Class	Label
1	Higher managerial, administrative and professional occupations
	1.1 Large employers and higher managerial and administrative occupations
	1.2 Higher professional occupations
2	Lower managerial, administrative and professional occupations
3	Intermediate occupations
4	Small employers and own account workers
5	Lower supervisory and technical occupations
6	Semi-routine occupations
7	Routine occupations
8	Never worked and long-term unemployed

Source: From Office for National Statistics, The National Statistics Socio-Economic Classification (NS-SEC rebased on the SOC2010). ©Crown copyright 2018. Office for National Statistics. Contains public sector information licensed under the Open Government Licence v3.0.

SOCIOLOGY

Higher classes also have the lowest refined carbohydrate intake. Adolescents from families in the lower social classes are more likely to snack on sugary items and these families tend to have higher caries rates and visit the dentist irregularly.

Psychological theories

There are various human psychological theories describing the stages of development and needs of an individual, such as Maslow's *hierarchy of needs* theory, which suggests that people are motivated to fulfil basic needs before moving on to other, more advanced needs.

The OHE might well come across these through wider reading, or when attending continuing professional development (CPD) meetings. They can be helpful when trying to understand a patient's responses and reaction to oral health instruction. Understanding how patients react differently to the same advice, and learning to modify your approach is part of reflective practice (see Chapter 16).

THE ICEBERG EFFECT

There is a difference between what the public perceive as their healthcare needs and their actual needs, which are determined by health professionals. This difference can be described by the *iceberg effect* (Figure 28.1). In this, differences in perception are not entirely the fault of the patient and can also be due to a lack of effective communication by the professional.

The dental professional's perceived need for treatment/action is represented by the whole iceberg, while the patient's knowledge (of what is needed) is represented by the tip of the iceberg. The four-fifths of the iceberg in between represents the *performance gap*, which is the difference between what professionals expect of patients and what some patients think is needed.

An example of the Iceberg Effect, experienced by the author, occurred when a dentist was showing a patient how to use Oral-B Superfloss™ around an implant, and the patient came out of the surgery asking the nurse how he would be able to do this with one hand. The nurse then showed him how to use an interdental brush.

Victim blaming

What the patient may see as responsible action, the health professional may see as irresponsible, especially if they are unaware of mitigating personal

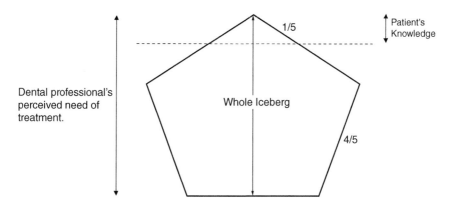

Figure 28.1 The iceberg effect. Source: From Ruth McIntosh. Reproduced with permission of Ruth McIntosh.

circumstances. This is known as *victim blaming* and can lead to the breakdown of dental professional/patient relationships.

The OHE is in a great position to reduce the performance gap and preserve the relationship, as shown in the following example.

An example of how to close the performance gap

The problem

The dentist suggests that a patient cleans their bridge interdentally daily with a well-known brand of interdental brushes. The patient cannot afford these brushes, but is too embarrassed to tell the dentist. Therefore, the bridge is not regularly cleaned, and dental problems occur. The dentist blames the patient for not acting on their advice, and the patient blames the dentist for not understanding their financial circumstances.

Negative result: the patient's oral health suffers, and they stop attending the practice.

The solution

Had an OHE been available when the bridge was fitted, the patient would have been more likely to reveal that the recommended interdental brushes were too expensive. The OHE could then help find a compromise, such as a less expensive alternative.

The OHE will have closed the performance gap using good communication and understanding, and ultimately lead to a positive, long-term professional/patient relationship.

SOCIOLOGY

REFERENCES

1. Ireland, R. (2004) *Advanced Dental Nursing*. Blackwell Science Ltd, Oxford.
2. Office for National Statistics (2010) *The National Statistics Socio-Economic Classification (NS-SEC rebased on the SOC2010)*. Available at: http://www.ons.gov. uk [accessed 25 September 2019].
3. The Health and Social Care Information Centre (2011) *Oral Health and Function – A Report from the Adult Dental Health Survey 2009*. The Health and Social Care Information Centre, Leeds.
4. NHS Digital (2015) *Child Dental Health Survey 2013, England, Wales and Northern Ireland*. Available at: https://digital.nhs.uk/data-and-information/publications/ statistical/children-s-dental-health-survey/child-dental-health-survey-2013-england- wales-and-northern-ireland [accessed 18 March 2019].

SOCIOLOGY

Chapter 29

Epidemiology

Learning outcomes

By the end of this chapter you should be able to:

1. Define *epidemiology* and explain why it is useful in dentistry.
2. State when UK dental surveys are conducted and explain how data is used.
3. List four terms frequently used in carrying out surveys.
4. Explain what an *index* is and be able to use different indices.

WHAT IS EPIDEMIOLOGY?

Epidemiology is the study of the distribution and determinants of health-related states or events (including disease), and the application of this study to control diseases and other health problems [1]. It is concerned with studying the presence of disease in a community, country or region, and can help to ascertain the size, severity, spread, and origin of a particular disease.

An epidemiologist deals with diseases and conditions in groups of people (whereas a clinician deals with those in individuals).

From epidemiological studies, decisions can be made on the allocation or targeting of resources in a given population. It is the foundation upon which governments and local authorities plan preventive measures for future generations, such as the fluoridation of water, or how many dentists will need to be trained in 20–30 years' time to meet demand.

The oral health educator (OHE) needs to know how dental surveys are used in epidemiology, as well as indices, which are used to measure data in populations and individuals.

Basic Guide to Oral Health Education and Promotion, Third Edition.
Alison Chapman and Simon H. Felton.
© 2021 John Wiley & Sons Ltd. Published 2021 by John Wiley & Sons Ltd.
Companion website: www.wiley.com/go/felton/oralhealth

SURVEYS

Surveys are systems used to collect and record data that is vital to epidemiology and the planning of future oral health.

Often, hundreds or thousands of subjects have to be surveyed, and the data must be recorded and analysed. Surveys must therefore be simple, reproducible, and not time-consuming.

As mentioned throughout this book, two surveys are of particular significance to the OHE in the UK:

- Adult Dental Health Survey (ADHS) 2009.
- Child Dental Health Survey (2013).

The main purposes of these surveys, which are carried out every 10 years, are to get a picture of the dental health of the population and how this has changed over time in order to assess changes in health and to plan for the future.

For example, some of the aims of the 2009 ADHS were to:

- Establish the condition of natural teeth and supporting tissues.
- Investigate dental experiences.
- Gain knowledge about attitudes towards dental care and oral hygiene.
- Examine changes in dental health over time.
- Monitor the extent to which dental health targets set by the government are being met.

For the ADHS, 11 380 individuals were interviewed, and 6 469 dentate adults were examined, making it the largest adult epidemiological survey ever in the UK.

The survey was commissioned by the NHS Information Centre for Health and Social Care, the Welsh Assembly Health Department, and the Department of Health, Social Services and Public Safety in Northern Ireland. It was managed principally by the Office for National Statistics (ONS). (Scotland did not participate.)

The 2009 survey consisted of a questionnaire interview for adults aged over 16 years at all sampled households, and an oral examination of the mouth and teeth of all those adults who had at least one natural tooth. Statistics were collected and recorded by community dental officers (often assisted by dental nurses), who examined sections of the population in their areas and charted the results.

These statistics were sent to the ONS where they were analysed, collated, and published in report form [2, 3]. Reports were then used by local authorities considering, for example, whether to fluoridate their water supply, or implement procedures to control drinks sold in school tuck shops.

Other surveys that may be of interest to those with a particular interest in epidemiology include national oral health surveys and publications from national health bulletins and personal communications that have been collated by The World Health Organization (WHO) into a database called CAPP [5].

Survey terminology

The OHE should be familiar with four terms that are used in the context of epidemiological surveys:

1. Screening – refers to examining the population.
2. Prevalence – looks at how widespread a condition is in the population.
3. Incidence – how often a condition occurs.
4. Distribution – assesses where most disease occurs in the population.

INDICES

An index (plural *indices*) is a numerical method of measuring data in a survey or in individuals.

Before indices were devised, oral hygiene and the extent of disease were graded by terms, such as *good, average,* or *poor*. Obviously, this was unsatisfactory as one person's idea of *good* may differ from another. Factors such as the extent of plaque and calculus were not recorded.

Examples of where indices can be used

Examples of data that can be gathered using indices include:

- Extent of caries – how many in a population are affected?
- Extent of periodontal disease – how widespread is it?
- Oral hygiene – how effectively are people cleaning teeth?
- Presence of plaque (or debris) – which surfaces are most commonly missed?
- Tooth loss – at what age do people most commonly lose teeth through gum disease?

There are many indices (especially for plaque), although the OHE need only have knowledge of those commonly used and in conjunction with a disclosing solution to measure the extent of plaque on the teeth. An OHE can use plaque and bleeding indices in education sessions to motivate patients, evaluate teaching, and may disclose mouths (with the patient's and dentist's permission) as long as they are trained to do so (see Chapter 31).

EPIDEMIOLOGY

DMFT caries index (1930s)

The DMFT (decayed, missing, filled teeth) index is the most commonly used index in UK epidemiological surveys of caries. It was developed by Klein and Palmer in the 1930s and the fact that it is still in use today indicates its success [4]. An important point to remember with this index is that large-case letters (DMFT) denote permanent teeth, while small-case letters (dmft) denote deciduous teeth.

By counting the number of decayed, missing and filled teeth, it is possible to assess the extent of caries in a population. If the DMFT-S (S = *surfaces decayed or filled*) is counted, the technique becomes even more specific. (Scores of 1–5 are used.)

For example, a dentist and a nurse survey a class of schoolchildren and records decayed, missing, and filled teeth. For children, a def(t) or def(s) index is used, where the 'e' stands for extracted deciduous teeth, rather than those that are exfoliated (fall out) naturally:

- A filled tooth scores 1.
- If surfaces filled are counted (e.g. a *three-surface filling*), the score for that tooth becomes 3.
- A tooth extracted because of caries scores 5 (five surfaces are missing).

Oral hygiene index (1960)

The oral hygiene index (OHI) was developed by Greene and Vermillion, and its original form was a combination of two indices: a calculus index and a debris index for every tooth.

They scored calculus as follows:

0 = None present.
1 = Supragingival calculus covering less than 1/3 of the tooth surface.
2 = Supragingival calculus covering 1/3 or 2/3 of the tooth surface and small amounts of subgingival calculus present.
3 = Supragingival calculus covering more than 2/3 of the tooth surface or continuous bands of subgingival calculus.

The same scoring system was used for debris (plaque/food) and extrinsic staining. However, this index proved to be too complex and time-consuming for general use, so Greene and Vermillion simplified it in 1964, facilitating its use in wider population groups. The resulting *simplified oral hygiene index* (OHI-S) selected only six tooth surfaces from different areas, as being representative of the whole mouth.

Silness and Löe plaque index (1964)

The patient is disclosed, and the presence of plaque noted as follows:

- Code 0 = No plaque deposits visible in the gingival area.
- Code 1 = Plaque deposits visible in the gingival area after disclosing.

Turesky plaque index (1970) (Figure 29.1)

This relatively simple method of measuring the presence of plaque offers a high level of sensitivity and is a useful patient motivation tool.

Instructions for using the Turesky index:

1. Disclose the patient.
2. Record buccal, labial, palatal, and lingual surfaces for each tooth (using the index that follows):

   0 = no plaque (Figure 29.2).

   1 = Separate flecks of plaque at cervical tooth margin (Figure 29.3).

   2 = Thin, continuous band of plaque (up to 1 mm) at cervical margin (Figure 29.4).

   3 = Band of plaque more than 1 mm wide but covering less than 1/3 of the crown (Figure 29.5).

   4 = Plaque covering at least 1/3 but less than 2/3 of the crown (Figure 29.6).

   5 = Plaque covering 2/3 or more of the crown (Figure 29.7).
3. Calculate the percentage of plaque present:

$$\frac{\text{Total score}\left(\text{upper and lower arch}\right)}{\text{Number of teeth}\times10}\times100$$

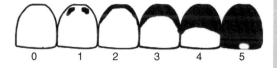

Figure 29.1 Turesky scores for plaque coverage. Source: Alison Chapman.

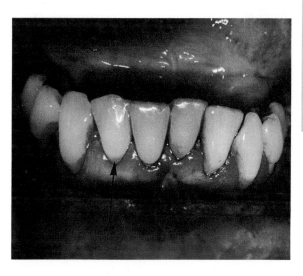

Figure 29.2 Turesky 0. Source: Alison Chapman.

EPIDEMIOLOGY

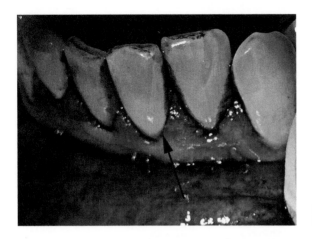

Figure 29.3 Turesky 1.
Source: Alison Chapman.

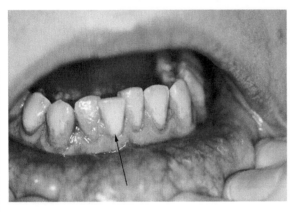

Figure 29.4 Turesky 2.
Source: Alison Chapman.

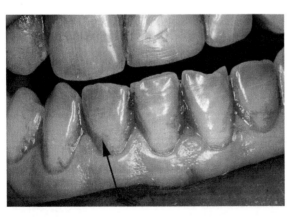

Figure 29.5 Turesky 3.
Source: Alison Chapman.

The OHE may not be able to look around the whole mouth, and if that is not possible, they should ask the dentist or dental hygienist to undertake this. The index can also be simplified to record the buccal surfaces only. Telling a patient that the percentage of plaque present can be a very good motivational

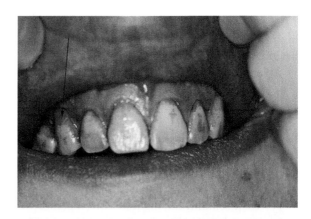

Figure 29.6 Turesky 4.
Source: Alison Chapman.

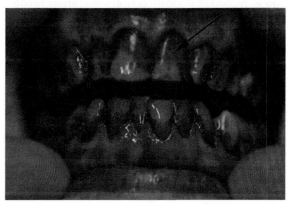

Figure 29.7 Turesky 5.
Source: Alison Chapman.

EPIDEMIOLOGY

tool by trying to reduce this at subsequent visits. It could also be used for healthy family rivalry!

Basic periodontal examination (BPE) index (1982)

OHEs do not carry out this examination, but may assist the dentist or hygienist by recording the data, and they can use the results to highlight areas of particular periodontal activity that the patient needs to address in their oral hygiene regime.

This screening system is based on the Community Periodontal Index of Treatment Needs (CPITN), which was developed by WHO in 1982, and subsequently adapted by the British Society of Periodontology (BSP).

For periodontal examination, the dentition is divided into six sextants. The WHO probe is recommended when undertaking this examination. It has a ball end 0.5 mm in diameter, and a colour-coded area which extends from 3.5–5.5 mm, and may also have a second colour-coded area running from 8.5–11.5 mm. Probing force should not exceed 20–25 g.

The probe tip is gently inserted into the gingival pocket and the depth of insertion read against the colour coding. The total extent of the pocket should be explored, by *walking* the probe around the pocket.

At least six points on each tooth should be examined:

- Mesiobuccal.
- Midbuccal.
- Distobuccal.
- Distopalatal.
- Midpalatal.
- Mesiopalatal (or lingual on lowers).

For each sextant, the highest score together with a '*' symbol (if appropriate) is recorded (Code * denotes furcation involvement). A sextant with only one tooth is recorded as missing (+) and the score is included in the adjacent sextant. A simple box is used to record the scores for each sextant.

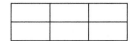

The BPE recording box

The following codes are used for diagnosis and treatment needs:

Code 0: Pockets 0–3 mm. Healthy gingivae with no bleeding on probing.

Treatment: no treatment required.

Code 1: Pockets 0–3.5 mm. Coloured area of probe remains completely visible in the deepest pocket in the sextant. No calculus or defective margins are detected. There is bleeding after probing.

Treatment: oral hygiene instruction (OHI).

Code 2: Pockets 0–3.5 mm. Coloured area of probe remains completely visible in the deepest pocket in the sextant. Supragingival or subgingival calculus is detected or the defective margin of a filling or crown.

Treatment: OHI plus removal of calculus and correction of plaque retentive margins of fillings or crowns.

Patients whose codes are 0, 1, and 2 should be screened annually.

Code 3: Pockets 3.5–5.5 mm. Coloured area of probe remains partially visible in the deepest pocket of the sextant.

Treatment: as per code 2, but more time will be required for treatment. Plaque and bleeding scores should be recorded at the start of the treatment and when the patient returns for an assessment visit after treatment is completed – usually 3 months.

Code 4: Pockets 5.5 mm and above. Coloured area of probe disappears into the pocket, indicating probing depths of at least 6 mm.

Treatment: a full probing depth chart is required together with bleeding and plaque indices, recession and furcation involvement, together with any other relevant clinical details. Individual intra-oral radiographs should be carried out for teeth with loss of attachment greater than 7 mm or furcation involvement.

Patients with 'code 4' and/or '*' should undergo a course of periodontal treatment including OHI, root surface debridement, and/or local or systemic antibiotic therapy as needed. This should be carried out by a suitably qualified person, such as a dental hygienist, a periodontist, or a dental practitioner with relevant experience.

Patients who have undergone a course of periodontal therapy should have full mouth charting repeated after a minimum of 3 months.

Children 12 years and younger
For children under 12 years old, only six index teeth are scored (they are all 6s; upper right 1 and lower left 1). Only codes 0, 1, or 2 are used because of the likelihood of false pocketing associated with newly erupting teeth. However, if the black band disappears into an unusually deep pocket, further investigation should be carried out and referral to a periodontal specialist considered.

REFERENCES

1. World Health Organization (2019) *Epidemiology*. Available at: www.who.int/topics/epidemiology/en/ [accessed 1 October 2019].
2. The Health and Social Care Information Centre (2011) *Oral Health and Function – A Report from the Adult Dental Health Survey 2009*. The Health and Social Care Information Centre, Leeds.
3. Office for National Statistics (2004) *2003 Dental Health Survey of Children and Young People*. Stationery Office Books, London.
4. Fejerskov, O. & Kidd, E. (2004) *Dental Caries: The Disease and Its Clinical Management*. Blackwell Munksgaard, Oxford.
5. World Health Organization (2019) *Oral health databases*. Available at: www.who.int/oral_health/databases/en/ [accessed 1 October 2019].

EPIDEMIOLOGY

Chapter 30

Evidence-based prevention

Learning outcomes

By the end of this chapter you should be able to:
1. Explain the meaning of the term *evidence-based prevention*.
2. Explain (giving examples) what is meant by the terms: *primary*, *secondary*, and *tertiary* prevention.
3. Show awareness of the Cochrane Collaboration and risk management in the practice.
4. State recommendations of the NICE report on dental attendance.
5. Be aware of the Dental Contract Reform Prototypes Scheme.

PREVENTION IS BETTER THAN CURE

Prevention is crucial in improving the general health of the nation, and in oral health it encompasses a wide range of strategies designed to prevent the development of dental diseases and conditions, which should ideally be initiated in early childhood.

Examples of prevention include:

- Fluoridation of drinking water (see Chapter 11).
- Administration of topical fluoride in toothpaste and by other means if thought necessary, such as tablets and drops for infants, mouthwash, gels, and varnish for older children and adults (see Chapters 11 and 14).
- Fissure sealing of first permanent molars (see Chapter 12).
- Choosing a diet low in simple sugars (see Chapter 10).
- Effective oral hygiene techniques (see Chapter 19).
- Regular dental check-ups – that screen for diseases and conditions, such as mouth cancer, caries, and periodontal disease.

Basic Guide to Oral Health Education and Promotion, Third Edition.
Alison Chapman and Simon H. Felton.
© 2021 John Wiley & Sons Ltd. Published 2021 by John Wiley & Sons Ltd.
Companion website: www.wiley.com/go/felton/oralhealth

EVIDENCE-BASED PREVENTION

The term *evidence-based prevention* is used when research has shown that a particular strategy in reducing dental disease has been effective. For example, it can be scientifically proven that the addition of fluoride to drinking water and toothpaste reduces caries, and there are studies linking the consumption of sugar to caries (see Chapter 5).

In the UK, great emphasis is placed on the importance of evidence-based prevention by the Department of Health and Public Health England (PHE), and the oral health educator (OHE) should be familiar with their key publication, *Delivering better oral health: an evidence-based toolkit for prevention* [1].

There are three main types of prevention: primary, secondary and tertiary.

Primary prevention

Primary prevention should be directed at healthy patients and aims to prevent illness and improve the quality of health and life, as all patients should be given the benefit of advice regarding their general and dental health, not just those thought to be at risk.

It is good practice to reiterate primary prevention to patients, even if they have good oral health, and to make sure they are aware of potential problems even if none currently exist (e.g. erosion from fizzy drinks, mouth cancer risks from smoking, and alcohol misuse). Patients may also pass on this advice to family members and friends.

Examples of primary prevention include:

- Fluoridation of drinking water.
- Advice to pregnant mothers and parents/guardians of small children on avoiding or reducing unnecessary sugars, and stressing the importance of brushing regularly with fluoride paste (see Chapter 21).
- Fissure sealing – first permanent molars before decay can develop.
- Advice to pre-teenage children on the dangers to the oral cavity of smoking, drinking alcohol, and taking drugs (see Chapter 13).

Secondary prevention

Secondary prevention is concerned with detecting a disease or condition early on and preventing it from further progression. It is particularly directed towards at-risk patients.

Examples of secondary prevention include helping patients towards:

- Resolution of gingivitis (particularly in the young). Simple oral health measures are applied to avoid progression to periodontitis (see Chapter 3).

- Remineralisation of early caries by using a fluoride toothpaste or GC Recaldent™ Tooth Mousse, and by modifying diet (see Chapter 9).
- Bringing children to the dentist for fillings whilst cavities are still small.
- Control of the dental manifestations of systemic diseases, e.g. diabetes (see Chapter 8).

Tertiary prevention

Tertiary prevention is directed at people who have a terminal or unresolvable condition or disability. It is aimed at improving the quality of life by limiting or delaying complications and, where possible, avoiding unnecessary hardships, restrictions and complications. Relatives and carers of patients in at-risk groups may also need help and advice (see Chapter 24).

Examples of tertiary dental health care include:

- Care of a crown or bridge (see Chapter 19).
- Care of partial or full dentures (see Chapter 23).
- Maintaining oral health when advanced periodontal disease is present.
- Care of the mouth when the patient has a medical condition that makes effective oral hygiene difficult.

The Cochrane Collaboration

Independent scientific evidence to support advice given to patients can be found on the *The Cochrane Collaboration* [2] website – a series of systematic reviews of primary research – originally established by Professor Archie Cochrane in the 1970s. Cochrane saw the need to establish an international network of groups, which would simplify evidence-based decision-making in clinical practice, and today the reviews are internationally recognised as the highest standard in evidence-based health care (see also Chapters 29 and 33).

Several organisations have been set up with the aim of standardising and integrating the methods used to develop guidelines for clinical practice, including the Scottish Intercollegiate Guidelines Network (SIGN).

EVIDENCE-BASED PREVENTION

RISK MANAGEMENT STRATEGIES

Ideally, each dental practice should have risk management strategies for prevention and clearly written policies, protocols, and procedures on the management of oral diseases, such as caries and periodontitis. This ensures that the whole dental team is working towards the same goals with regard to patient treatment and advice.

NICE recommendations on patient recall

In 2004, the National Institute for Clinical Excellence (NICE) produced a guide on how often dentists should carry out routine check-ups, and practices still find the document useful in determining recall intervals for patients. Much scientific literature was reviewed in order to assess risks to patients if (6-monthly) dental check-ups were carried out less frequently.

The findings were as follows [3]:

- There is little need for 6-monthly check-ups over any other frequency of recall.
- Shortening the interval to less than 6 months results in small reductions in caries, but not other conditions.
- Changes are determined by individual risk (patients' needs may vary).
- Making the interval between check-ups longer than 6 months is more cost-effective.
- NICE also suggested that reviews for patients on the basis of disease risk assessments should be undertaken between:
  - 3–24 months (for adults).
  - 3–12 months (for children).

The dental professional (usually the dentist) has the responsibility to use their clinical judgement when determining the interval between check-ups, but should consult the patient (or carer, if applicable) when making the decision.

While many patients who have good general and oral health are fine on an annual check-up, some need more interventions. For example, many older patients have multiple heavily filled teeth and/or are taking many medications, and so they have more frequent problems that, if left, could seriously affect their oral health. Also, many young children are still experiencing tooth decay despite advice and treatment.

DENTAL CONTRACT REFORM: PROTOTYPES SCHEME

At the time of writing, a pilot of 102 NHS practices is taking part in the Dental Prototype Agreement Scheme, which is testing new ways of trying to drive oral health improvement through prevention, aiming to [4]:

- Prevent future dental disease.
- Encourage patients to take responsibility for their oral health, with the support of the practice team.
- Reduce the amount of necessary remedial dental work.

EVIDENCE-BASED PREVENTION

The scheme uses a clinical pathway that gives patients oral health assessments that [4]:

- Identify the patient's future risk of dental disease.
- Provide self-care plans and preventative advice.

Follow-up *Oral Health Reviews* are provided where necessary, and patients also still have access to the full range of NHS clinical treatments.

REFERENCES

1. Public Health England and Department of Health (2017) *Delivering better oral health: an evidence-based toolkit for prevention (third edition)*. Available at: www.gov.uk/government/publications/delivering-better-oral-health-an-evidence-based-toolkit-for-prevention [accessed 30 April 2019].
2. The Cochrane Collaboration (2019) *Cochrane Reviews*. Available at: www.cochrane.org/search/site/cochrane%20reviews [accessed 2 October 2019].
3. National Institute for Health and Care Excellence (2004) *Dental checks: intervals between oral health reviews Clinical guideline [CG19]*. Available at: www.nice.org.uk/guidance/CG19 [accessed 3 October 2019].
4. Department of Health and Social Care (2018) *NHS dental prototype agreements: patient information*. Available at: www.gov.uk/government/publications/nhs-dental-prototype-agreements-patient-information [accessed 3 October 2019].

EVIDENCE-BASED PREVENTION

Chapter 31

UK dental services

Learning outcomes

By the end of this chapter you should be able to:
1. Explain the roles of the National Health Service (NHS) and private practices in dentistry.
2. Explain what is meant by *clinical governance*, with reference to the *Donabedian concept*.
3. Describe the ways in which the public can obtain dental treatment.
4. Explain the role of the General Dental Council (GDC) in relation to the dental team and oral health educators (OHEs) in particular.

NHS DENTAL SERVICE

The NHS was set up in 1948 with the aim of providing free medical and dental treatment for the whole population, regardless of social status. Funded by the government from taxation, it soon became the envy of the world.

Over the years, there have inevitably been many changes to the NHS, including the provision of dental care. Perhaps, the most significant change has been that adults have had to pay increasingly towards the costs of NHS dental treatment. However, pregnant/nursing mothers, children in full-time education, and those receiving certain benefits and allowances are still entitled to free dental treatment.

Basic Guide to Oral Health Education and Promotion, Third Edition.
Alison Chapman and Simon H. Felton.
© 2021 John Wiley & Sons Ltd. Published 2021 by John Wiley & Sons Ltd.
Companion website: www.wiley.com/go/felton/oralhealth

PRIVATE DENTAL PRACTICES

In 1990, the government made radical changes to the way NHS dentists were paid and as a result many dentists left the NHS and adopted private schemes. Such schemes are not liked by all patients, and some private practices still continue to provide free treatment for exempt groups. Cost became a major factor in discouraging certain population groups from attending.

REVIEW OF NHS DENTAL SERVICES IN ENGLAND

In 2009, the Department of Health appointed an independent group to review NHS dentistry, led by Professor Jimmy Steele [1].

The subsequent report stressed the need to make the transition from dental activity to oral health as the outcome for the NHS dental service, and set out a framework for care. Its publication initiated a new impetus for NHS dentistry based on evidence-based care pathways, and has resulted in prototype studies involving NHS practices, which could well shape the future of NHS dental care and access to high-quality services (see Chapter 30).

THE HEALTH AND SOCIAL CARE ACT 2012

The Health and Social Care Act 2012 has been perhaps the most significant change to the NHS since its inception and was designed to meet the healthcare challenges of the future by making the NHS more responsive, efficient, and accountable.

The Act places clinicians in charge of shaping services to enable NHS funding to be spent more effectively. For example, in England most NHS services are now commissioned by clinical commissioning groups (CCGs) for their populations, which play a key role in driving up the quality of primary medical care locally, being responsible for approximately 60% of the NHS budget. NHS England work with, and support, CCGs and hold them to account for improving outcomes for patients, and in getting the best value-for-money from public investment. This is done at local level by regional teams. NHS England also provides guidance and tools, based on the best available evidence, to enable them to commission effectively, and pick up those services it would not be possible or appropriate for CCGs to commission, including dentistry.

The Act also enables patients to choose services that best meet their needs from 'Any Qualified Provider', including charitable or independent sector providers, as long as they meet NHS costs. Providers, including NHS foundation trusts, are free to innovate to deliver services.

CLINICAL GOVERNANCE AND DONABEDIAN'S MODEL

In 1969, Avedis Donabedian, Professor of Public Health in Michigan (USA), developed a conceptual model for examining health services and evaluating the quality of healthcare given, which is regarded by many professionals worldwide as having transformed the way healthcare was delivered.

Donabedian's concept was one of the theories which led to clinical governance and quality control in dental practices and trusts, including: requirements for staff to have appropriate and recognised qualifications, continuing professional development (CPD), and practice inspections to ensure that equipment is up-to-date and conforms to health and safety regulations.

Clinical governance was introduced to the NHS in 1998 and was designed to bring a systematic approach to the delivery of high-quality healthcare. Private practices are also required to comply with the requirements of quality control.

Donabedian's three principles

Donabedian's model stated that the assessment of the quality of care should be based on three principles [2]:

1. Structure.
2. Process.
3. Outcome.

These principles when applied to providing quality dental care can be expanded as:

- Structure – provision of facilities (e.g. surgery access, equipment), and organisation of the practice (e.g. staff training, qualifications and CPD, patient/staff ratio, personnel attributes).
- Process – what the dentist and team do in the delivery of care for patients, including:
  - Taking and regularly updating medical histories.
  - Delivering excellent treatment.
  - Attention to health and safety of patients and staff at all times.
- Outcome – producing evidence that shows that patients are:
  - Satisfied with the quality of care (e.g. via short questionnaires, when they return for routine check-ups).
  - Offering to redo any treatment which has fallen short of patients' expectations free of charge.

UK DENTAL SERVICES

- Developing good relationships with patients so that they feel they can complain if not satisfied.
- Ensure that complaints or suggestions will be followed up promptly.

THE GENERAL DENTAL COUNCIL

The General Dental Council (GDC) is the organisation that regulates dentists and other dental care professionals (DCPs) in the UK. Its main purpose is to protect the public by regulating the dental team, and the organisation consults the views of the public, patients, and registrants when making policy and decisions.

All dentists and other DCPs (including dental nurses, dental technicians, dental hygienists, dental therapists, and orthodontic therapists) must be registered with the GDC [3]. Individuals must be able to demonstrate certain outcomes by the end of their training in order to register as a dental professional and member of the dental team. All DCPs must also show continuing professional development (CPD) and record it during 5-year cycles. The GDC keeps records of each DCP's CPD and can ask to inspect proof of undertaking.

The GDC expects all dental professional registrants to follow its *Scope of Practice and* uphold its *Standards for the Dental Team*.

GDC *Preparing for practice*

The GDC's Preparing for practice document [4] describes the outcomes that a dental professional must be able to demonstrate in order to be registered with the GDC. The OHE should be familiar with these extensive outcomes and be able to carry them out in relation to oral health education and promotion (as well as their other duties).

Briefly, the outcomes are:

- Clinical – e.g. be able to explain the causes and development of caries and periodontal disease.
- Communication – e.g. effectively communicate information and provide reassurance on oral hygiene products to patients and their representatives.
- Professionalism – e.g. to be able to recognise/respect a patient's perspective and expectations.
- Management and Leadership – e.g. taking responsibility for their personal development, recording evidence, and reflective practice.

GDC Scope of Practice

The GDC's Scope of Practice details the skills and abilities that dental nurses and other registered DCPs should have, and includes a list of all tasks that the professional can do. The GDC continually reviews the *Scope of Practice* to incorporate changes/advances in dentistry. At present, patients must be seen by a dentist before being treated by any other member of the dental team (with the exception of dental technicians in certain cases, and dental hygienists), but this may change in the future.

The Scope of Practice also includes additional skills that the professional can develop post registration to increase their scope of practice and expand/ deepen one's knowledge in a particular area, including oral health and promotion for dental nurses: *'Additional skills dental nurses could develop include: further skills in oral health education and oral health promotion'* [3].

However, dental nurses must not carry out procedures in the oral cavity that constitute the *practice of dentistry*. This is a *grey area*, but is generally taken to mean that no dental instrument should be used by a dental nurse within the mouth. OHEs are advised to seek permission from their employer and the patient before demonstrating toothbrushing/flossing and other procedures within the mouth. (Some dentists train nurses to use a probe in the mouth in order to show patients where they have missed plaque.)

If dentists are uncertain about what procedures a nurse/OHE may carry out, they should seek advice from their dental indemnity company. With registration, nurses are required to provide their own indemnity and can therefore consult their own company if asked to carry out procedures for patients that they are unsure about.

GDC Standards

The GDC Standards [5] sets out nine principles that each member of the dental team should adhere to, and a failure to do so, can result in being removed from the GDC register and unable to work as a dental professional.

Under the Standards for the Dental Team [5]:

- *'You must only carry out a task or a type of treatment if you are appropriately trained, competent, confident and indemnified. Training can take many different forms. You must be sure that you have undertaken training which is appropriate for you and equips you with the appropriate knowledge and skills to perform a task safely.'*
- *'You should only deliver treatment and care if you are confident that you have had the necessary training and are competent to do so. If you are not confident to provide treatment, you must refer the patient to an appropriately trained colleague.'*

CARE QUALITY COMMISSION

The Care Quality Commission (CQC) is England's health and social care regulator. As part of its remit it regulates all primary dental care services – both private and NHS – and publishes up-to-date information from its assessments.

UK DENTAL SERVICES

While clinical governance looks at the people looking after patients and makes sure their skills are always up-to-date, the CQC looks at the way the practice is run and that conditions are safe for patients. It assesses and inspects health and social care environments, publishes reports on whether national standards are met, and welcomes patients sharing their experiences with them.

In Wales, Care Inspectorate Wales (CIW) register, inspect and take action to improve the quality and safety of services for the wellbeing of the population. In Scotland, the health care regulator is the Care Inspectorate, and the regulation of the private health care sector comes under Healthcare Improvement Scotland (HIS). In Northern Ireland, the Regulation and Quality Improvement Authority (RQIA) is the independent body responsible for monitoring and inspecting the availability and quality of health and social care services, and encouraging improvements in the quality of provision.

COMMUNITY DENTAL SERVICE

The Community Dental Service (CDS) in England provides specialist dental services to patients in the community: for those individuals who have difficulty in getting treatment in dental practices and who require treatment on a referral basis, which is not available in a general dental care setting. For example, community dental professionals look after young children who need special help, as well as housebound people and those with severe physical disabilities or mental illness.

Community dental care workers treat people in their own homes, and in residential and nursing homes (known as *domiciliary care*) if they are unable to attend a surgery. They work with a wider clinical team including other DCPs and health professionals, such as school nurses, health visitors, and district nurses.

In Wales, Community Dental Services (CDS) provide treatment for people who may not otherwise seek or receive dental care, such as those with learning disabilities, the elderly, housebound people, and those with mental or physical health problems that prevent them from visiting a dentist.

In Northern Ireland, the Community Dental Service is a group of dental practitioners providing a wide range of specialist dental services in health centres and hospitals to people with special care needs.

In Scotland, the Public Dental Service is responsible for treating patients with special needs or patients requiring specialised services, including surgical dentistry and paedodontics, as well as services for anxious patients (including sedation and general anaesthetics).

HOSPITAL DENTAL SERVICES

In university dental hospitals, patients are treated by students as part of their training (supervised by qualified personnel). General dental practitioners (GDPs) can refer patients to specialised clinics within hospitals for the diagnosis and treatment of oral diseases that are not treatable in general practice, but there may be long waiting lists for procedures other than emergencies.

Cases treated include advanced periodontal disease, mouth cancer, orthodontics and other specialisms, such as maxillofacial trauma and facial deformity (e.g. cleft lip and/or palate – usually picked up through the hospital service after birth).

Patients can also be seen by dental students for routine examinations and treatment if they are not registered with a dentist. An advantage of this service is that there is no fee. However, as mentioned, treatment may take much longer than in general practice and the patient must be available for long appointments.

REFERENCES

1. Department of Health (2009) *NHS Dental Services in England, An Independent Review Led by Professor Jimmy Steele.* Department of Health, London.
2. Donabedian, A. (2005) Evaluating the Quality of Medical Care. *The Milbank Quarterly.* 83, 691–729.
3. General Dental Council (2013) *Scope of Practice.* Available at: www.gdc-uk.org/docs/default-source/scope-of-practice/scope-of-practice.pdf?sfvrsn=8f417ca8_4 [accessed 20 December 2019].
4. General Dental Council (2015) *Preparing for practice – Dental team learning outcomes for registration.* Available at: https://www.gdc-uk.org/docs/default-source/quality-assurance/preparing-for-practice-(revised-2015).pdf?sfvrsn=81d58c49_2 [accessed 20 December 2019].
5. General Dental Council (2013) *Standards for Dental Professionals.* Available at: https://standards.gdc-uk.org/ [accessed 20 December 2019].

UK DENTAL SERVICES

Chapter 32

Oral health promotion

Learning outcomes

By the end of this chapter you should be able to:
1. Distinguish between *oral health promotion* and *oral health education*.
2. Be aware of local/national/global programmes and initiatives, and how to get involved.
3. Be aware of Department of Health guidance on *Delivering better oral health*.
4. Explain barriers to promotion.

WHAT IS ORAL HEALTH PROMOTION?

It is important for oral health educators (OHEs) to know the difference between oral health education and promotion.

Oral health education is part of the wider aspect of oral health promotion, which involves policy-driven local, national, and international programmes and initiatives, which either target the population directly or are communicated via educators.

According to the World Health Organization (WHO) [1]: *'Health promotion policy combines diverse but complementary approaches including legislation, fiscal measures, taxation and organizational change. It is a coordinated effort towards creating supportive environments and strengthening community action. Health promotion works through concrete and effective community actions in setting priorities, making decisions, planning strategies and implementing them to achieve better health.'*

Basic Guide to Oral Health Education and Promotion, Third Edition.
Alison Chapman and Simon H. Felton.
© 2021 John Wiley & Sons Ltd. Published 2021 by John Wiley & Sons Ltd.
Companion website: www.wiley.com/go/felton/oralhealth

DEFINING PEOPLE'S NEEDS

If oral health promotion is to be effective, it is necessary to define people's *needs* rather than *wants*. For example, the population *needs* fluoridated water – the British Dental Association (BDA) recommends it, the House of Lords has endorsed it, but large groups within communities still object to it, and so it cannot be implemented.

Epidemiological surveys (see Chapter 29) show that people in poorer, deprived areas suffer greater dental disease than those in more prosperous areas and the needs expressed by people in poorer areas are more likely to be free treatment, rather than water fluoridation. This is known as *felt need*, and should be taken into account when professionals are assessing what they call *normative need* (the measures that they know will improve oral health).

The overall aim of oral health promotion is to influence the social norms of a community towards change and improvement through evidence-based prevention (e.g. water fluoridation, smoking cessation). Greatest benefit will ultimately be obtained by combining *high-risk* approaches (where groups or individuals thought to be at highest risk of disease are targeted), with the population approach (such as water fluoridation).

INTERNATIONAL ORAL HEALTH PROMOTION

The Ottawa Charter

In 1986, WHO produced a document called *The Ottawa Charter*, which is an example of an international health promotion initiative.

The Charter is an international agreement that was signed at the First International Conference on Health Promotion in Ottawa (Canada). It set in motion a series of research studies and initiatives among international organisations, national governments, and local communities to achieve a goal of *Health for All* by the year 2000, and better health promotion beyond.

Strategies in the Charter included [2]:

- Building healthy public policy (e.g. legislation exempting toothpaste from VAT, adding fluoride to water).
- Local authority healthy eating policies.
- Creating supported environments (putting policies into action by making the healthy choices easy).
- Developing individual knowledge and skills in those who deal with the public, including doctors, dental personnel, pharmacists, caterers, teachers, and nursery staff.

ORAL HEALTH PROMOTION

- Supporting community action – working with voluntary groups to care for the health in their communities.
- Re-orientating health services towards prevention and ensuring that all health professionals give the same message.

WHO's Global Oral Health Programme

Building upon the Ottawa Charter, WHO's current Global Oral Health Programme is geared towards disease prevention and health promotion through evidence-based strategies. The Organization places great emphasis on developing policies in promotion and prevention to help build healthy populations worldwide and combat poor health; focusing on changing behaviours related to diet, nutrition, tobacco, excessive alcohol consumption, and hygiene. This is set out in the following strategies [3]:

- 'Reducing oral disease burden and disability, especially in poor and marginalized populations.
- Promoting healthy lifestyles and reducing risk factors to oral health that arise from environmental, economic, social, and behavioural causes.
- Developing oral health systems that equitably improve oral health outcomes, respond to people's legitimate demands, and are financially fair.
- Framing policies in oral health, based on integration of oral health into national and community health programmes, and promoting oral health as an effective dimension for development policy of society.'

Within these strategies, emphasis is placed on stimulating the community-oriented projects for the oral health promotion and prevention of oral diseases, by translating evidence into action programmes at community or national levels (see following text). They place a high priority on improving the oral health of the elderly and children.

WHO oral health priority action areas

The Global Oral Health Programme focuses on the following priority action areas [3]:

- Risks to oral health and intervention:
  - Diet, nutrition, and oral health – which affects oral health in many ways.
  - Oral health and fluoride – in caries prevention.
  - Tobacco and oral health – particularly in young people and women in developing countries.
- Important target areas:
  - School children and youth – e.g. WHO's Global *School Health Initiative*, which aims to mobilise/strengthen health promotion and education activities at local/national/regional/global level, such as the *Health promoting school* (HPS); '*one that constantly strengthens its capacity as a healthy setting for living, learning and working*' [3].

- Elderly people – with the proportion of older people rising.
- HIV/AIDS and oral health – contributions to the early diagnosis, prevention, and treatment of oral manifestations of this disease.
- Oral health services – ensure availability/access to essential high-quality health services, especially in deprived communities.
- Information systems – provide public healthcare administrators and decision-makers with the tools, capacity, and information to assess and monitor health needs in order to choose intervention strategies, design policy options, and improve the performance of the oral health system.

WHO public health recommendations (see Chapter 10)

WHO also publishes public health solutions for addressing caries through policy measures (which includes promotional measures to reduce free sugar consumption), such as [4]:

- Clear nutritional labelling.
- Improving the food environment in public institutions (e.g. schools, hospitals,
- work).
- Increasing awareness/access to safe, clean drinking water.

UK NATIONALLY-LED ORAL HEALTH PROMOTION INITIATIVES

The OHE should be aware of the national health promotion initiatives instigated and run by various organizations, including the Department of Health, the NHS, and charities.

The following text includes some of the main services, events, and publications, but you will no doubt be able to think of others, including your own perhaps?

Oral health promotion services

The OHE can signpost patients to services that promote oral (and general) health, including:

- NHS Stop Smoking Service (see Chapter 13).
- Alcoholics Anonymous (see Chapter 13).

Annual promotion events

The OHE can get involved with national (and worldwide) health and oral health specific promotion events, by either launching their own initiatives in line with the events, or by becoming involved in an existing initiative with other health professionals.

ORAL HEALTH PROMOTION

Regular annual health promotion events include:

- *Alcohol Awareness Week* – run each November by Alcohol Change UK.
- *BNF Healthy Eating Week* – run each June by the British Nutritional Foundation (BNF)
- *Dry January* – run each January by Alcohol Change UK.
- *Mouth Cancer Month* – run each November, supported by the Mouth Cancer Foundation and the British Dental Health Foundation.
- *National No Smoking Day* – takes place on the second Wednesday in March each year and funded by government and voluntary organisations.
- *National Smile Month* – run each May by the Oral Health Foundation.
- *Nutrition and Hydration Week* – run in March by a group of organisations.
- *Stoptober* – run each October by Public Health England (PHE).
- *World Cancer Day* – 4th February, run by the Union for International Cancer Control (UICC).
- *World Health Day* – each April, run by WHO.
- *World Oral Health Day (WOHD)* – run on the 20th March each year by the FDI World Dental Federation.

Promotion publications

There are many examples of oral health promotional publications (including leaflets and posters), that the OHE can utilise. Examples include:

- *Smoke Free and smiling: helping patients to quit tobacco* (*a Department of Health Publication*) (see Chapter 13).
- *Mouth Heroes for Schools: helping teachers give lessons on good oral health* (an FDI World Dental Federation publication) [5].
- *Toolkit for Sports Organizations* (an FDI World Dental Federation publication) [6].
- *Dental Buddy and schools* (Oral Health Foundation) – resources for delivering oral health in the classroom [7].

Department of health guidance

In 2005, the UK Department of Health produced a guidance document entitled *Choosing Better Oral Health, An Oral Health Plan for England*, which was sent to all NHS dental practices to help promote oral health in patients through dentists and other dental care professionals (DCPs). It is an example of a national oral health promotion initiative.

In 2007, this was superseded by a document called *Delivering Better Oral Health: An Evidence-Based Toolkit for Prevention*, which was also delivered to all NHS dental practices by the Department of Health. A subsequent second edition (2009) and third edition (2017) were sent to all dental practices to provide essential guidance for dentists and DCPs [8].

ORAL HEALTH PROMOTION

The Toolkit sets out, in considerable detail, guidance on improving oral health through evidence-based research. It is essential that oral health education students and practitioners thoroughly familiarise themselves with this document and use this promotional tool to deliver educational messages.

GETTING INVOLVED WITH LOCAL ORAL HEALTH PROMOTION INITIATIVES

Many national health promotion services will have local branches, such as the NHS Stop Smoking Service and Alcoholics Anonymous, which the OHE can *signpost* patients towards.

As mentioned, the OHE can also become part of national events (which may well have regional or local initiatives as part of them). However, the OHE should also be aware of other local health promotion activities specific to their community that they can become involved with – *grass roots* promotion – which can be just as effective in promoting healthy lifestyles.

The enthusiastic educator can also set up their own promotion initiatives, such as schemes to give talks, workshops, and exhibitions in schools, residential homes, and community centres (see Chapter 18).

BARRIERS TO PROMOTION

As with oral health education, some people respond to promotion, but others do not, and no matter how strong the argument for a particular promotional initiative, there are certain people (and groups) who are extremely reluctant to engage.

The reasons behind this reluctance are complex and involve many factors, including:

- Community reasons – e.g. local resistance to water fluoridation.
- Social factors – conforming to perceived social norms (see Chapter 28).
- Economic reasons – e.g. unable to afford good quality food or oral hygiene products.
- Lack of knowledge/skills – people cannot change their behaviour unless they have the education and knowledge to do so.
- Some population groups do not visit dental professionals regularly, or ever.

ORAL HEALTH PROMOTION

FUTURE PROMOTION

Fifty years ago, many adults would have expected to lose many, if not all, of their teeth by middle age, and treatment was aimed at cure rather than prevention. However, the most recent surveys of adult dental health (2009) and child dental health (2013) show that the oral health of the nation is improving, which is due in part to developments in oral health education and promotion [9,10]. However, there are still regional and cultural variations and there is much still to be achieved.

OHEs should never underestimate their ability or the impact they have in improving patients' health and lives, and the future of oral health promotion is a particularly exciting area of expertise, with new initiatives and pilot schemes based on evidence-based prevention under way (see Chapter 31).

Outside of the practice, health promotion is endemic in all our lives, and there will be many more opportunities for the OHE to become involved and play an increasingly significant part in this dynamic field.

REFERENCES

1. The Ottawa Charter for Health Promotion First International Conference on Health Promotion, Ottawa, 21 November 1986.
2. Ireland, R. (2004) *Advanced Dental Nursing*. Blackwell Science Ltd, Oxford.
3. World Health Organization (2019) *Oral health*. Available at: www.who.int/health-topics/oral-health/#tab=tab_1 [accessed 16 October 2019].
4. World Health Organization (2017) *Sugars and dental caries – WHO Technical Information Note*. Available at: www.who.int/oral_health/publications/sugars-dental-caries-keyfacts/en/ [accessed 20 March 2019].
5. Public Health England and Department of Health (2017) *Delivering better oral health: an evidence-based toolkit for prevention (third edition)*. Available at: www.gov.uk/government/publications/delivering-better-oral-health-an-evidence-based-toolkit-for-prevention [accessed 30 April 2019].
6. FDI World Dental Federation (2019) *Mouth Heroes for Schools: helping teachers give lessons on good oral health*. Available at: https://www.fdiworlddental.org/news/20190403/mouth-heroes-for-schools-helping-teachers-give-lessons-on-good-oral-health [accessed 10 March 2020].
7. FDI World Dental Federation (2019) *Toolkit for Sports Organizations (Sports Dentistry)*. Available at: https://www.fdiworlddental.org/resources/toolkits/toolkit-for-sports-organizations [accessed 10 March 2020].
8. Oral Health Foundation (2018) *Dental Buddy and schools*. Available at: https://www.dentalhealth.org/Pages/FAQs/Category/downloads [accessed 10 March 2020].

ORAL HEALTH PROMOTION

9. The Health and Social Care Information Centre (2011) *Oral Health and Function – A Report from the Adult Dental Health Survey 2009*. The Health and Social Care Information Centre, Leeds.
10. NHS Digital (2015) *Child Dental Health Survey 2013, England, Wales and Northern Ireland*. Available at: https://digital.nhs.uk/data-and-information/publications/statistical/children-s-dental-health-survey/child-dental-health-survey-2013-england-wales-and-northern-ireland [accessed 18 March 2019].

Chapter 33
Dental research

Learning outcomes

By the end of this chapter you should be able to:
1. Understand scientific terminology used in research papers.
2. Describe the facets of a clinical trial.
3. Source research papers in journals and on the Internet.

KEEPING UP TO DATE WITH RESEARCH

The field of dentistry is forever changing and the oral health educator (OHE) should keep up to date with the latest scientific research that is relevant to education and promotion. This can be done by reading and understanding research papers and studies as part of their continuing professional development (CPD). Research papers can be obtained by reading journals and searching the Internet.

Research findings can be interesting, but it is also necessary to be able to interpret the way that it has been carried out to decide whether the results are clinically significant. The OHE should also ascertain how the research was funded and if there may be bias. For example, if it was funded by a commercial company who could benefit from the results?

Significance of research papers

When the OHE reads a research paper, a structured approach will help decide upon its significance to their role, by considering:

- What is the specific aim of the study?
- What are the outcomes?

Basic Guide to Oral Health Education and Promotion, Third Edition.
Alison Chapman and Simon H. Felton.
© 2021 John Wiley & Sons Ltd. Published 2021 by John Wiley & Sons Ltd.
Companion website: www.wiley.com/go/felton/oralhealth

- How was the study conducted?
- How good is the evidence?

Terminology

When looking at a research paper, the terminology used can appear complex. However, becoming familiar with the following scientific terms should help the OHE find their way through.

Abstract

An abstract is a brief overview of a study/piece of research, which includes the subject, principle tools used, results, and conclusions.

Qualitative research

Qualitative research is used to explore and understand people's beliefs, experiences, attitudes, behaviour, and interactions. For example, to record opinions in focus groups.

Quantitative research

Quantitative research generates numerical data or data that can be converted into numbers, such as clinical trials or the National Census. For example: '8 out of 10 people questioned said they flossed daily'.

Epidemiology

Epidemiology is the study of the distribution and determinants of disease within a population. Commonly, the findings are reported for the benefit of public health (see Chapter 29).

Incidence

Incidence describes the occurrence, rate, or frequency of new diseases (such as periodontal disease, heart disease, or cancer) in a defined population over a specific period of time.

Prevalence

Prevalence describes the total number of existing cases, during a particular period of time (*period prevalence*) or at a particular date in time (*point prevalence*).

Control group

A control group (sometimes just referred to as the *control*) refers to a group of subjects in a trial, where the factor being tested is not applied. A control group therefore serves as a standard for comparison against other experimental groups where the factor is applied.

DENTAL RESEARCH

For example, in the Vipeholm Study (see Chapter 5) the control group ate a normal diet when conducting experiments with sugar in the study of the incidence of caries. This can also be applied when work is carried out *in vitro* (see later in Chapter), where prepared samples are set aside and used to measure differences with those samples that have undergone an experiment.

Cross-sectional study

A cross-sectional study involves data collected from a representative sample of a population in order to estimate the point prevalence of disease.

Case-control study

A case-control study is one that looks back (retrospectively) at two groups of people. One group has a condition (*case*), the other group (*control*) does not. Researchers can assess how many people were exposed to a certain risk factor to see if that had an effect on their health.

For example, a study could be looking at a group who have lung cancer and a group who do not. They would then see how many people in each group smoked in order to ascertain whether there could be a link between lung cancer and smoking.

Cohort study

A cohort is a term for *a group of people with a shared characteristic.*

Cohort studies look at the experiences of a sample of the population having a certain type of treatment, or of being exposed to certain risk or beneficial factors. A study will comprise an exposed group and a control group. Unlike a case-control study, a cohort study looks forward (prospective) rather than backwards (retrospective).

An example of a cohort study would be one looking into any potential differences in caries rates between two groups of people: one group that lives in a fluoridated water area and another group who does not. Such studies often take years to complete.

Matching

Matching is a technique used by researchers in studies to try and make the results as reliable as possible. Researchers may try to match cases and controls for a variety of general factors, such as age, gender, and lifestyle (e.g. alcohol consumption and smoking history).

In situ research

In situ research is that which is conducted to examine a phenomenon that takes place exactly where it occurs. For example, wearing oral appliances with enamel samples that can be investigated in their natural environment.

DENTAL RESEARCH

In vitro research

In vitro research is that which is conducted in an artificial environment (usually in the laboratory), using components of an organism (also known as *test-tube* experiments).

In vivo research

In vivo research is that which is conducted in a living organism, such as humans and rats.

CLINICAL TRIALS

A clinical trial is a particular type of clinical research that involves patients, and/or healthy people. Clinical trials follow a set of rules (protocols) to ensure that they are as safe and as accurate as possible. The more clinical trials conducted on a study, the more robust the findings.

Clinical trials help determine whether:

- Treatments are safe.
- Treatments have any side effects.
- New treatments are better than current treatments.

There are different types of studies that can be used in clinical trials, including: randomised controlled, cohort, single or double blind, crossover and parallel studies.

Randomised controlled trial/study

In a randomised controlled trial, participants are randomly allocated to a group, one of which will act as a control group that may receive a placebo treatment (containing no active ingredient).

A minimum of two groups are required (one treatment-based, the other placebo), and each group is exposed to a different procedure/element. Participants are closely monitored, and the results recorded over a specific length of time. These are then used to assess the trial results.

Cohort study

See *Terminology*.

Single-blind and double-blind studies

In a single-blind study, either the participants or observers/investigators are unaware of the intervention being carried out. In a double-blind study, both the investigators and the participants are unaware of the intervention being carried out.

DENTAL RESEARCH

Crossover study

Crossover studies look at factors that are thought to increase the risk of a particular outcome in the short term. In a crossover study, each participant is involved in the different interventions, and preferably in a random order. The interventions will usually be separated by an amount of time or *wash-out* period.

Parallel study

In a parallel study, two groups are subjected to different interventions at the same time, unlike a crossover study in which participants take part in all interventions.

SOURCING RESEARCH PAPERS

The following sources of research papers can be found on the Internet and/or in print, and will be of use to the OHE (as well as other health professionals):

- British Association of Dental Nurses (BADN).
- British Association for Oral and Dental Research (BSODR).
- British Dental Journal (BDJ).
- British Society of Dental Hygiene and Therapy (BSDHT).
- Cochrane UK.
- Department of Health and Social Care (DHSC).
- Evidence-Based Dentistry (EBD).
- European Journal of Oral Science.
- Google Scholar.
- International Association for Dental Research (IADR).
- Journal of Dentistry.
- Journal of Evidence-Based Dental Practice.
- National Institute for Health and Clinical Excellence (NICE).
- National Oral Health Promotion Group (NOHPG).
- PubMed.
- Science Direct.
- The American Dental Association (ADA).

These databases and journals are easily found by typing in their names into a search engine, but be aware that some websites charge for their services.

The OHE can also ask professional colleagues for help when trying to find clinical papers and in acquiring printed publications, as well as contacting dental training establishments for permission to use their library facilities.

DENTAL RESEARCH

Index

Note: Tables and figures are indicated by an italic *t* and *f* following the page number.

Basic Guide to Oral Health Education and Promotion, Third Edition.
Alison Chapman and Simon H. Felton.
© 2021 John Wiley & Sons Ltd. Published 2021 by John Wiley & Sons Ltd.
Companion website: www.wiley.com/go/felton/oralhealth